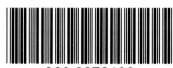

An Atlas of
PROSTATIC DISEASES
Third edition

THE ENCYCLOPEDIA OF VISUAL MEDICINE SERIES

An Atlas of
PROSTATIC DISEASES
Third edition

Roger S. Kirby, MD, FRCS(Urol), FEBU

Professor of Urology

St. George's Hospital

London, UK

The Parthenon Publishing Group

International Publishers in Medicine, Science & Technology

A CRC PRESS COMPANY

BOCA RATON   LONDON   NEW YORK   WASHINGTON, D.C.

Published in the USA by
The Parthenon Publishing Group Inc.
345 Park Avenue South, 10th Floor
New York
NY 10010
USA

Published in the UK and Europe by
The Parthenon Publishing Group
23–25 Blades Court
Deodar Road
London SW15 2NU
UK

Library of Congress Cataloging-in-Publication Data
Data available on application

British Library Cataloguing in Publication Data
Kirby, R.S. (Roger S.)
  An atlas of prostatic diseases. - 3rd ed. - (The
  encyclopedia of visual medicine series)
  1. Prostate - Diseases - Atlases
  I. Title
  616.6'5

ISBN 1-84214-216-X

First published in 2003

Composition by The Parthenon Publishing Group
Printed and bound by T. G. Hostench S.A., Spain

Contents

Preface

A picture, it has been said, is worth a thousand words. In this third edition of the *Atlas of Prostatic Diseases*, I have tried to tell the story of the prostate in images and illustrations rather than words, keeping the text pithy and very focused. In this busy information world, none of us has time to plough through dense and lengthy tomes; instead, all of us prefer to come straight to the point. Succinctness is what I have tried to achieve here. In today's world, less is more.

In the two previous editions, I concentrated on the causes, diagnosis and staging of prostate cancer, benign prostatic hyperplasia and prostatitis. These have all been updated for this third edition. Furthermore, I have added a new section on treatment of these three very common conditions, with algorithms to summarize the decision-making processes for each of them at various stages of each disease. I have tried to make this as up-to-date as possible, adding, for example, the latest data from the Medical Therapy of Prostate Symptoms (MTOPS) study. I have also included some of the latest information about some new strategies for the management of the thorny problem of androgen-independent prostate cancer.

The prostate, and the diseases to which it is prone, has recently become the focus of intense media interest and frequent debate. Men's health in general has suddenly become a major public health issue. I hope that this new edition of the Atlas will help both to inform the debate and to educate the urologists, family physicians and nurse practitioners about the prostatic diseases and related disorders that impact negatively on the quality of life of so many men.

Finally, I would like to thank Dee McLean who has worked so hard to produce the illustrations.

Roger S. Kirby
St. George's Hospital, London

I

Introduction

Recently, the prostate gland has emerged from the shadows into the full glare of media publicity; these days, barely a week goes by without the feature of some high-profile sufferer of prostate disease in the media. What lies behind this surge of interest? Prostate problems are increasingly common and men are now more inclined than ever before to discuss and debate them. Rising life expectancy has swollen the ranks of men of middle age and beyond. These individuals have a 43% risk of symptoms of benign prostatic hyperplasia and a 9% chance of being diagnosed as suffering from prostate cancer. Prostatitis, the third component of the triad of diseases considered in this Atlas, ranks among the 20 most frequent causes of outpatient visits to urologists, and is a cause of significant morbidity among sufferers.

Although not always life-threatening, prostate diseases are often associated with a significant reduction in quality of life not only for the sufferer, but also for his partner. The ever-swelling numbers of men beyond middle age are increasingly reluctant to accept restrictions on their day-to-day activities as they grow older. For the first time, an effective lobby is developing, both in the United States and in parts of Europe, to press governments, insurers and health-care providers for a more active approach to prostate disease. Prostate diseases are now acknowledged as an important determinant of men's health and therefore worthy of proper scrutiny and enhanced research effort.

In this volume, the anatomy and physiology of the normal prostate are described. The molecular basis and pathology of benign prostatic hyperplasia, prostate cancer and prostatitis are illustrated. The Atlas concludes with a description of the means of diagnosis and ever-evolving modalities of treatment for these very troublesome and highly prevalent disorders.

2

Anatomy and embryology

The lobar concept of the anatomy of the prostate originally suggested by Lowsley[1] is no longer particularly helpful. The accepted view today is that of McNeal[2], who suggested that the prostate consists of three distinct zones: a central zone, transitional zone, and peripheral zone (Figures 1 and 2). The transitional zone is the site of development of benign prostatic hyperplasia, whereas the peripheral zone is where both prostatitis and prostate cancer mainly occur[3].

The explanation for these contrasting zonal susceptibilities to different diseases probably lies in their different phylogenetic origins. In primates, the gland is divided into a cranial prostate and a caudal prostate (Figure 3). Their fusion in humans creates a single gland that completely encircles the urethra, but the different zonal pathological tendencies underline their disparate origins.

EMBRYOLOGICAL DEVELOPMENT OF THE PROSTATE

In the developing fetus, the urogenital sinus begins to divide the cloaca by around day 28 of gestation

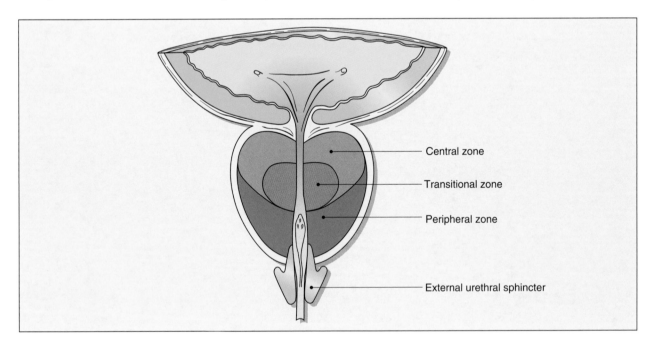

Figure 1   The prostate is composed of three distinct zones: the peripheral zone; the transitional zone; and the central zone (anteroposterior view). Prostate cancer most commonly originates in the peripheral zone; in contrast, benign prostatic hyperplasia almost exclusively affects the transitional zone and periurethral tissues

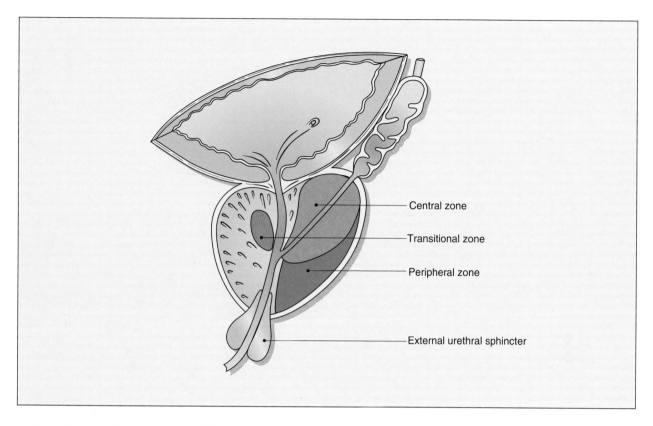

Figure 2   The three zones of the prostate (sagittal view)

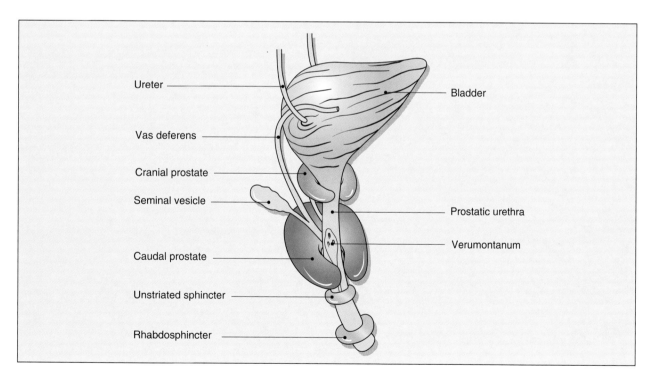

Figure 3   In primates, the prostate is divided into a caudal prostate and a cranial prostate. In phylogenetic terms, the cranial prostate is thought to be the precursor of the central zone whereas the caudal prostate is considered the precursor of the peripheral zone. In humans, the two structures are fused, but the zones are susceptible to different disease processes

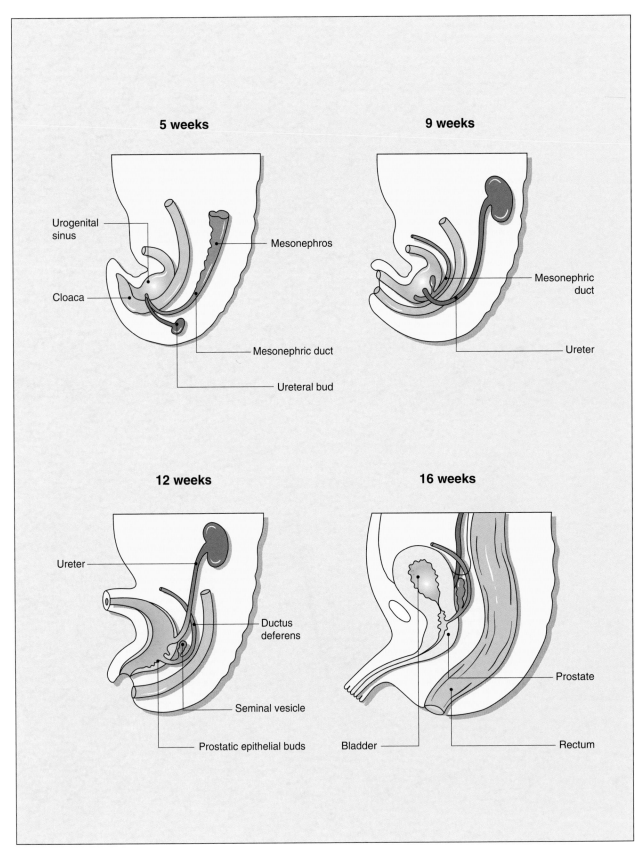

Figure 4 Embryology of the prostate: the gland develops at the base of the bladder as outgrowths from the urethra and coalesce with the surrounding mesenchyme. This interaction forms the basis of the adult gland, which comprises a mixture of epithelium and stroma

(Figure 4). Both the rectum and the urogenital sinus can be recognized as separate entities by day 44 of embryonic development. The primitive urogenital sinus proximal to the mesonephric duct is destined to become the vesicourethral canal; in contrast, the region distal to the mesonephric duct develops into the definitive urogenital sinus.

The Müllerian tubercle is situated within the urogenital sinus just distal to the mesonephric (Wolffian) ducts, which are formed at an earlier stage of development. The Wolffian ducts eventually become the paired vasa deferentia and seminal vesicles. By day 28, the ureteric buds begin to sprout from the lower ends of the Wolffian ducts; the ureters subsequently separate completely to merge into the trigonal tissue which is developing cranially.

Subsequent to this division of the primitive cloaca, the prostate itself begins its morphogenesis during the 12th week of intrauterine growth. Multiple endodermal outgrowths appear from the epithelial lining of the prostatic portion of the urogenital sinus and rapidly insinuate themselves into the surrounding mesenchyme. These prostatic ducts soon lengthen and branch, and eventually canalize to form distinct glandular structures. The stimulus for this development appears to be testosterone secreted from the developing testes and, of crucial importance, its more potent 5α-reduced dihydrotestosterone (DHT) metabolite, produced within the gland by the enzyme 5α-reductase. As discussed below, the genomic mutations that result in a congenital absence of this enzyme in the fetus lead to failure of the prostate and external genitalia to develop and a reduced susceptibility to neoplasia.

Prostatic glandular epithelium becomes differentiated from invaginated cells, and mesenchymal cells eventually develop into the interposing stroma, which consists of both smooth muscle cells and fibroblasts. The interaction through cell-to-cell signalling between stromal and epithelial cells underlies not only this process of differentiation, but also the growth disorders that constitute both the benign prostatic hyperplasia and prostate cancer that frequently beset men beyond middle age.

ANATOMY OF THE PROSTATIC DUCTS

In humans, the prostate is composed of approximately 20 branching glandular structures, which spread out into a matrix of fibromuscular stroma (Figure 5). Current evidence suggests that newly formed epithelial cells are mainly located in the distal segments of the glands. In the mid-acinar

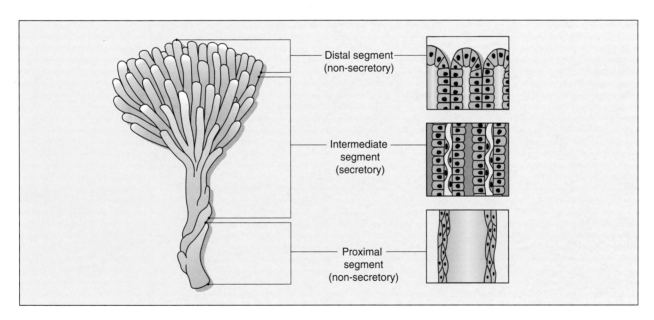

Figure 5   Prostatic ducts arborize throughout the gland and terminate in acini which secrete, among other things, prostate-specific antigen (PSA) into the lumina and thence into the prostatic urethra. New cells are formed in the distal segments of the ducts, whereas the intermediate section is secretory in function. In the proximal segment, epithelial cells become flattened and undergo programmed cell death (apoptosis)

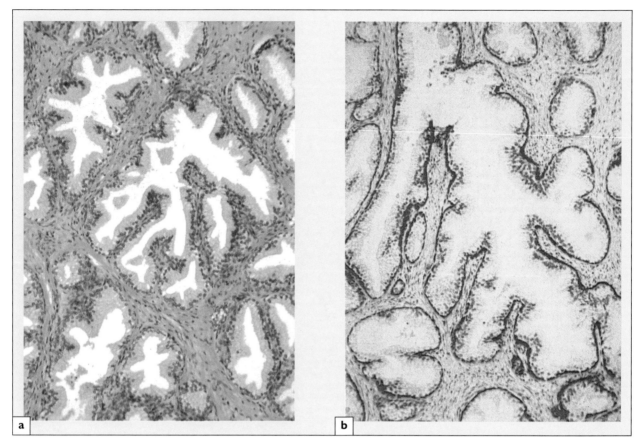

Figure 6   Normal prostatic acini are lined by tall columnar cells with a peripheral basal cell layer (a; H & E). The latter cell layer is more easily seen when stained immunocytochemically by antibody CK 5+6 against cytokeratins of high molecular weight (b)

portions, epithelial cells are tall and columnar, and perform a secretory role (Figure 6). In the distal ductal portions, the epithelial cells are lower in height and exhibit frequent apoptosis (programmed cell death).

The major function of prostatic epithelium is to elaborate and secrete prostate-specific antigen (PSA; Figure 7). Discovered by Wang and colleagues[4], PSA is a single-chain glycoprotein consisting of 237 amino acids. The gene encoding PSA is located on chromosome 19, close to the androgen response element (ARE). Transcription of this gene is stimulated by the formation of intracellular DHT. Messenger RNA (mRNA) encoding PSA is then translated into a glycoprotein protease (of the kallikrein family). The role of PSA is to liquefy semen after ejaculation and thereby to release spermatozoa to migrate within the female genital tract.

Normally, only a small proportion (< 0.1%) of the total PSA output is absorbed across the basal cell layer and through the basement membrane into the bloodstream; normal serum levels are usually below 4 ng/ml (Figure 8). In the bloodstream, as one might expect of an active protease, the majority of PSA is bound to protein, either antichymotrypsin or α_2-macroglobulin. A proportion of PSA remains unbound or 'free'.

However, prostatic diseases, especially prostate cancer, which result in damage to the integrity of the basal cell layer and basement membrane, are associated with PSA levels greater than this value; thus, PSA is able to serve as a marker for pathological changes[5]. In addition, increasing age in itself is associated with gradual progressive PSA elevation[6] (Figure 9), perhaps due to increasing leakage of PSA across the basement membrane or due to developing benign prostatic hyperplasia. For reasons that are unclear, in men with prostate cancer the amount of free (unbound) PSA is reduced. The ratio of free to total PSA can therefore be helpful in deciding who

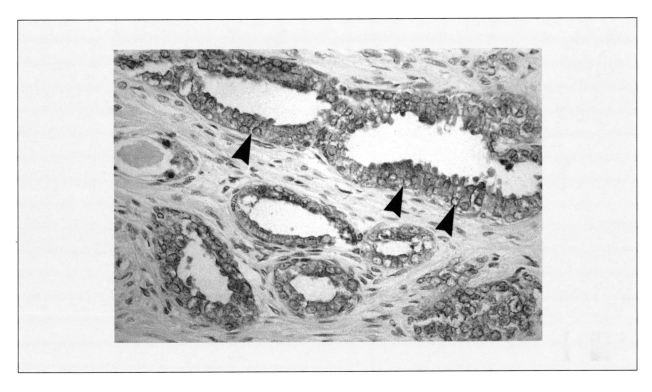

Figure 7   Prostate-specific antigen (PSA) can be demonstrated in luminal cells by immunocytochemical staining. The basal cells (arrowed) can be shown not to contain PSA

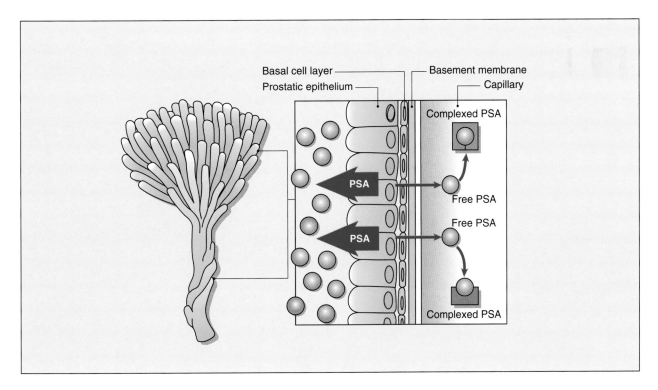

Figure 8   Prostate-specific antigen (PSA) is a glycoprotein protease secreted by the epithelium of prostatic acini. Most of the PSA produced eventually reaches the ejaculate wherein its function is to liquefy semen. Around 0.1% of the total volume, however, is absorbed across the basement membrane to reach the bloodstream, where it is mainly bound by either antichymotrypsin or α_2-macroglobulin

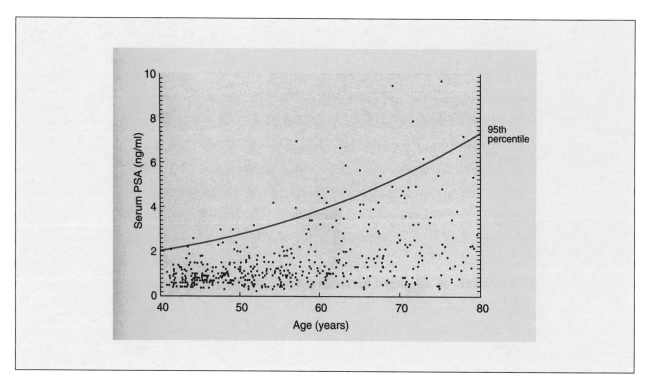

Figure 9   Probably as a result of age-associated leakiness of the basal cell layer and basement membrane, but also because of benign prostatic hyperplasia, serum prostate-specific antigen (PSA) values tend to increase with age

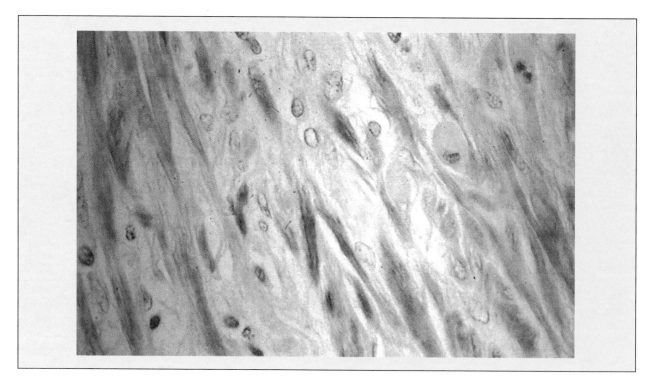

Figure 10   A considerable proportion of the prostate is composed of stroma rather than epithelium, the dominant constituent of which is smooth muscle cells, as exemplified by this section of normal prostate (immunocytochemical preparation)

should or should not undergo prostate biopsy to exclude malignancy.

STROMAL-TO-EPITHELIAL RATIOS

The ratios of stroma to epithelium in the normal and hyperplastic prostate have been studied quantitatively by both Bartsch and colleagues[7] and Shapiro and colleagues[8]. Morphometric data suggest that the normal prostate is composed of approximately 40% smooth muscle (Figure 10) and 20% glandular epithelium. In benign prostatic hyperplasia, particularly that of the stromal variety, the smooth muscle component may be as much as 60% of the total volume (Figure 11). Between individuals, however, there is wide variation, with marked tissue heterogeneity even within the same gland.

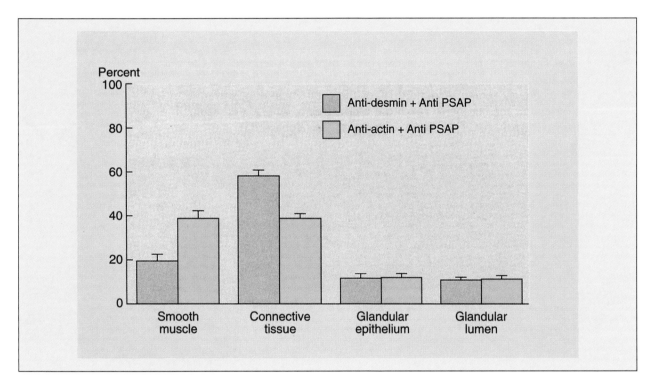

Figure 11   The ratio of stroma to epithelium in the human prostate, as calculated by Shapiro and colleagues[8]. In some patients with benign prostatic hyperplasia, the preponderance of stroma over epithelium increases even further, to up to 60% of total prostate volume

3

Innervation of the prostate

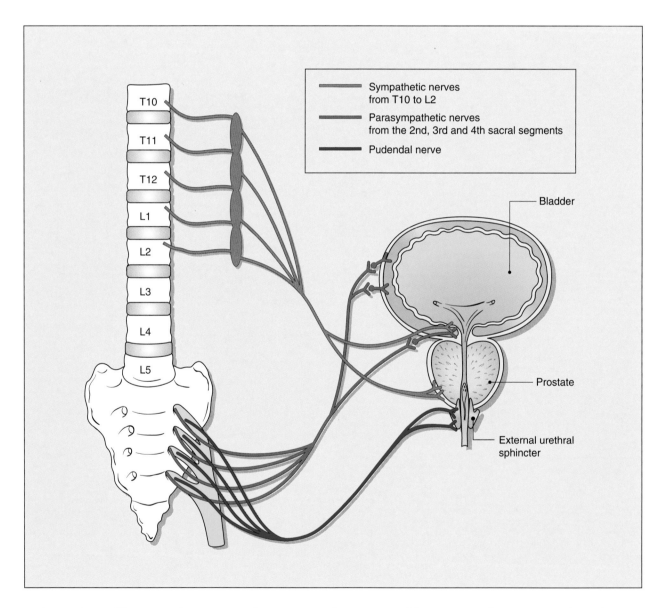

Figure 12   Three sets of nerves control continence and micturition. The parasympathetic system induces detrusor contraction during voiding, whereas the sympathetic nerves and the pudendals (somatic) maintain prostatic and urethral muscle tone in order to maintain continence

To explain the innervation of the prostate, it is necessary to describe briefly the neurophysiology of continence and micturition. The bladder and urethra are innervated by three sets of nerves: the sympathetic, from T10 to L2 spinal levels, the parasympathetic, from sacral spinal segments S2 to S4, and the pudendal nerve, which carries somatic innervation from S2 to S4 (Figure 12).

During bladder filling, sensory nerve endings detect progressive stretching of the bladder wall and convey information via the parasympathetic nerves to the spinal cord and brain. Increasing activity in these nerves produces a progressive reflex contraction in the bladder neck and prostatic urethra, as well as in the external urethral sphincter, thereby maintaining urinary continence.

When the bladder volume reaches 300–500 ml, an awareness of the need to void develops, although true bladder contractions should not occur until a socially convenient time arrives. Voluntary voiding is accomplished as a result of a barrage of impulses down the parasympathetic nerves to the detrusor muscle (Figure 13). The neurotransmitter acetylcholine is released, which binds to muscarinic receptors on detrusor smooth muscle cells to produce coordinated contraction of the bladder body.

At the same time, neural impulses passing down the sympathetic and pudendal motor fibers cease momentarily, thereby allowing relaxation of the normally tonically contracted, continent bladder neck, prostatic urethra and external sphincter. Bladder pressure rises, the bladder neck funnels and urine flow commences, achieving a maximum flow rate of more than 15 ml/s, with a maximum detrusor pressure of less than 40 cmH$_2$O.

Provided that the urethra is unobstructed, bladder contraction continues until emptying is complete; urethral and bladder neck tonus is then re-established and the bladder-filling cycle begins again.

The main functional innervation of the prostate is through the sympathetic (noradrenergic) nervous system (Figure 14), although acetylcholinesterase-containing (presumably parasympathetic) and non-adrenergic, non-cholinergic nerve fibers are also present.

Intraneural recordings from peripheral nerves elsewhere in the body reveal continuous waves of motor impulses from small, unmyelinated, so-called C fibers, which subserve tonic vasomotor tone. Presumably, a similar situation occurs within the prostate; it has been proposed that bladder outflow obstruction due to benign prostatic hyperplasia may be related to chronic overactivity of the sympathetic nervous system, in the same way that chronic overactivity of vasomotor fibers may result in systemic hypertension.

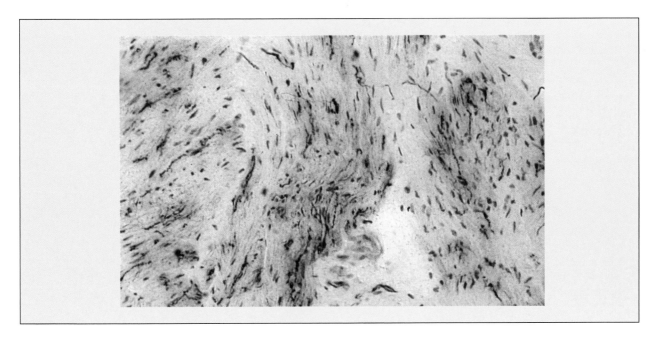

Figure 13   The parasympathetic innervation of the detrusor muscle can be demonstrated by use of a special stain for acetylcholinesterase. Nerve fibers are stained brown and can be seen in association with the detrusor smooth muscle cells

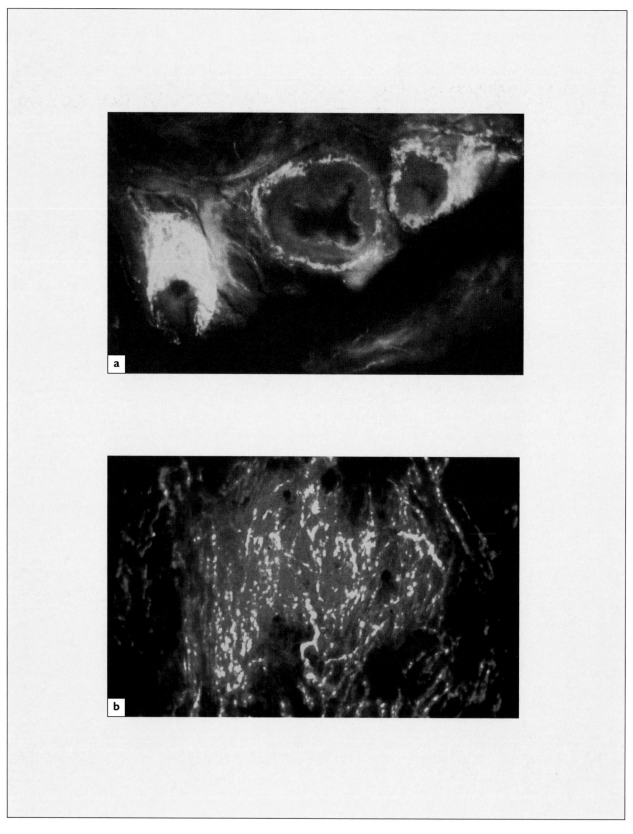

Figure 14   Immunofluorescent staining of sympathetic nerve endings in the wall of a blood vessel (a). These nerves are responsible for the maintenance of vasconstrictor tone. Catecholamine immunofluorescence staining demonstrates the rich sympathetic innervaton of the prostate (b). Sympathetic nerves control prostatic smooth muscle tone and can be modulated by α_1-adrenoceptor blockers

4

Ejaculatory function

Apart from its important role in maintaining urinary continence, prostatic and bladder neck sympathetic innervation is also essential for ejaculation. Erectile function, by contrast, is subserved by parasympathetic fibers, which pass in the so-called neurovascular bundles of Walsh lying posterolateral to the prostate; these fibers are capable of producing vasodilatation within the corpora cavernosa[9] (Figure 15). In this periprostatic location, these nerves are vulnerable to injury during either radical prostatectomy or radical cystoprostatectomy performed for the surgical excision of urological malignancy (Figure 16).

At the time of ejaculation, a synchronized sequence of sympathetically induced contractions develops in the vasa deferentia, seminal vesicles and

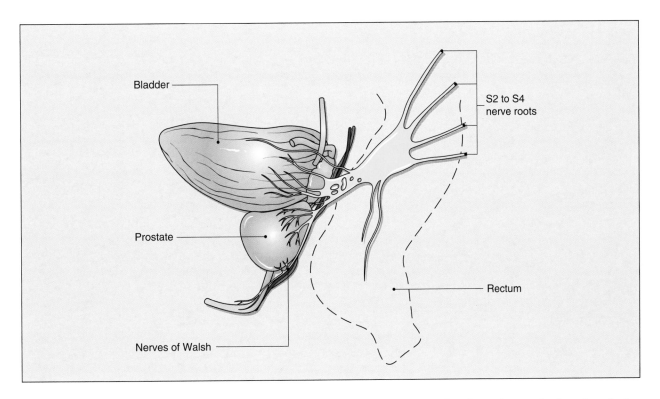

Figure 15   The neurovascular bundles, also known as the nerves of Walsh after the urologist who first described them, convey nerve impulses and blood to the corpora cavernosa and thereby subserve penile erection. Their location posterolateral to the prostate renders them vulnerable during radical prostatectomy or cystoprostatectomy

prostatic smooth muscle itself. This activity delivers a mixture of fluid from the seminal vesicles, semen from the vasa and fluid containing PSA from the prostate into the prostatic urethra, via openings in the verumontanum. Tight closure of the bladder neck then creates a 'pressure chamber' within the prostate such that, when reflex relaxation of the external sphincter occurs in conjunction with

pulsatile contractions of the bulbocavernous muscles, antegrade ejaculation results (Figure 17).

Prostatic surgical procedures, such as transurethral resection of the prostate or open prostatectomy, which render the bladder neck incompetent, interfere with this pressure chamber effect and consequently result in irreversible retrograde ejaculation.

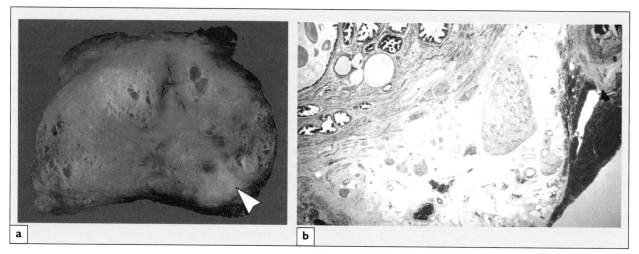

Figure 16 (a) Transverse section from a radical prostatectomy specimen. The cancer is located posteriorly (arrowed). (b) On histology, the neurovascular bundles can be seen lying posterolaterally, where they are susceptible to malignant infiltration. Prostatic intraepithelial neoplasia is present, but cancer is not seen at this level (H & E)

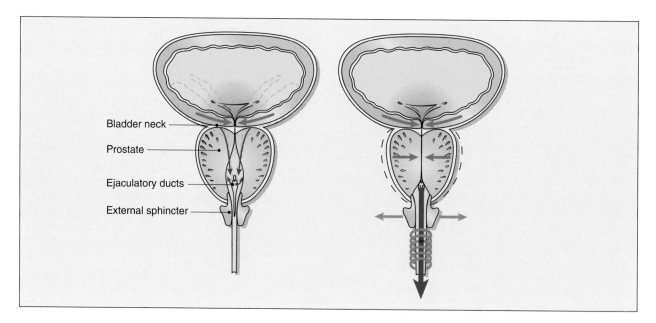

Figure 17 The mechanism of ejaculation is a complex neurophysiological process which involves contraction of the prostate and seminal vesicles, which empty their contents into the prostatic urethra. At the same time, the bladder neck closes to create a 'pressure chamber'. Rhythmic relaxation of the distal urethral sphincter and contractions of the bulbocavernous muscles around the bulbar urethra result in a pulsatile antegrade expulsion of a mixture of seminal and prostatic fluid

5

Molecular mechanisms underlying prostate growth

The prostate develops and grows under the controlling influence of the hypothalamo–pituitary axis (Figure 18). The hypothalamus normally secretes the decapeptide luteinizing hormone releasing hormone (LHRH) in a pulsatile fashion, which then passes down the pituitary stalk to the pituitary gland to provoke the release of luteinizing hormone (LH). LH enters the circulation and acts on the Leydig cells of the testes, thereby stimulating testosterone formation and release. Testosterone in the circulation is

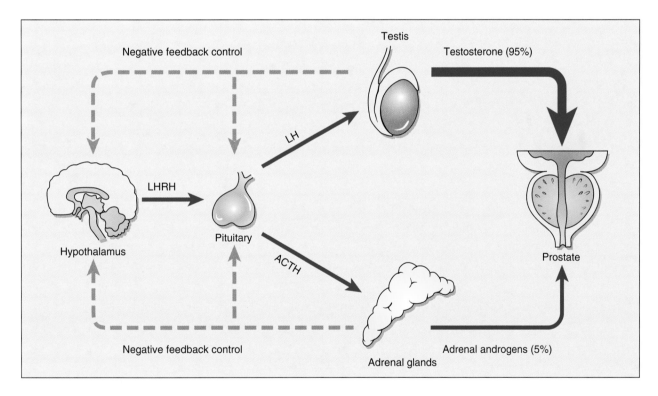

Figure 18   Growth and development of the prostate are under endocrine control. Luteinizing hormone releasing hormone (LHRH) is secreted by the hypothalamus and passes down the pituitary stalk to stimulate the pituitary itself to release luteinizing hormone (LH). LH in turn acts on the Leydig cells of the testis to induce secretion of testosterone (T), which stimulates prostatic growth. In addition, adrenocorticotrophic hormone (ACTH) induces secretion of weak androgens, such as androstenediol, from the adrenal cortex. These adrenal androgens provide approximately 5% of the androgen drive to the prostate in the healthy subject, but may acquire greater importance after orchiectomy or administration of LHRH analogs

mainly bound to sex hormone binding globulin (SHBG); only the unbound portion is available, to enter the cytoplasm and nucleus of prostatic cells by a process of simple diffusion.

In addition to testicular testosterone, a further 5% or so of circulating androgens is derived from the adrenal glands under the stimulatory influence of adrenocorticotrophic hormone. In health, the effects of these adrenal androgens, mainly in the form of androstenedione and androstenediol, are relatively insignificant. However, these adrenal androgens assume some importance after chemical or surgical castration because they remain in the circulation and may, after conversion to DHT within the prostate, stimulate continuing growth and division of prostate cancer cells.

Once inside a prostate cell, testosterone is rapidly metabolized by the enzyme 5α-reductase, located on the nuclear membrane, to DHT[10,11]. It is this 5α-reduced form of testosterone that binds with the androgen receptor. The process of DHT binding involves the release of so-called heat-shock protein (hsp 90) and the dimerization, together with conformational change, of paired androgen receptor structures (Figure 19).

Thus, a segment of deoxyribonucleic acid (DNA) within the genome of the prostate cell initiates DNA transcription, producing mRNA, which encodes, among other cytokine molecules, epidermal growth factor (EGF) and platelet-derived growth factor (PdGF). These growth factors, in turn, stimulate prostate cell growth by specifically activating growth factor receptors located on the cell membrane of epithelial and stromal cells[12] (Figure 20).

In the normal prostate, growth homeostasis is achieved by a balance between release of growth stimulating factors, such as EGF and PdGF, and growth inhibitors, such as transforming growth factor-β (TGF-β). TGF-β not only inhibits cell

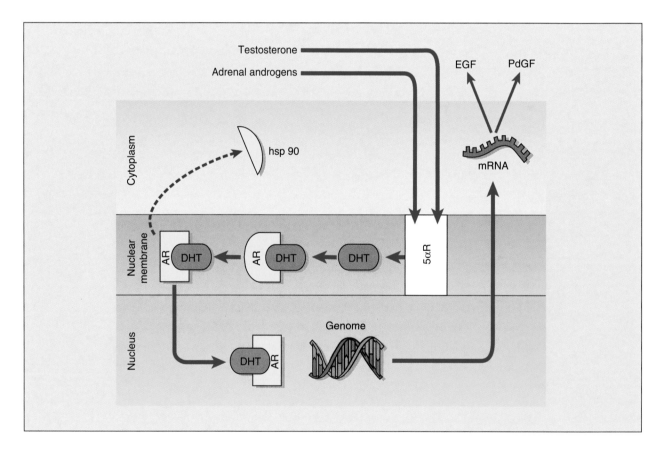

Figure 19   Testosterone enters prostatic cells by simple diffusion. The enzyme 5α-reductase (5αR) type II, which is located on the nuclear membrane, metabolizes testosterone to dihydrotestosterone (DHT), a more active androgen. DHT then binds to the androgen receptor (AR) of the genome that releases heat-shock protein 90 (hsp 90) and stimulates the transcription of androgen-inducible genes, including growth factors such as epidermal growth factor (EGF) and platelet-derived growth factor (PdGF)

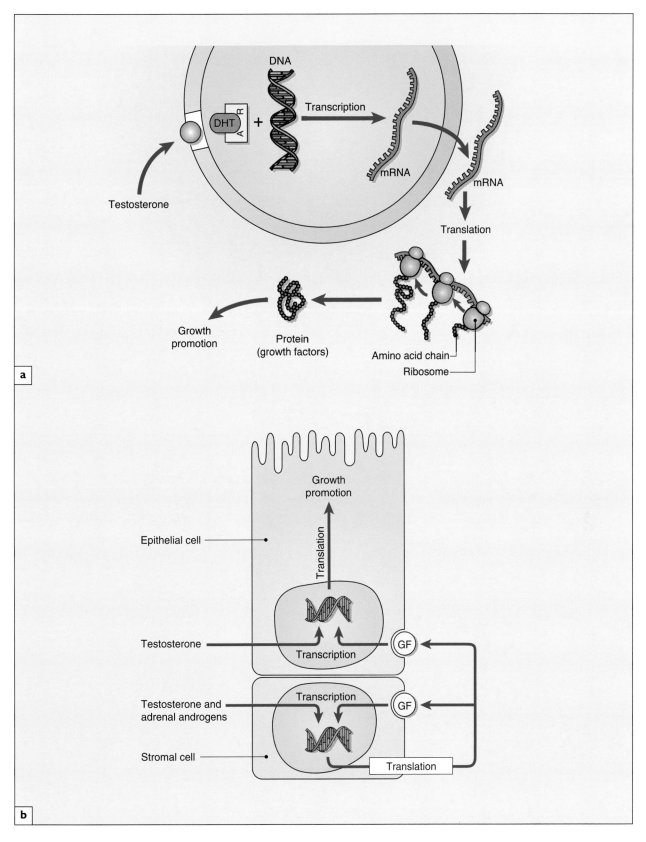

Figure 20   (a) Following androgen stimulation of the genome, messenger ribonucleic acid (mRNA) is produced and translated into the specific protein sequences that encode growth factors, such as epidermal growth factor and platelet-derived growth factor. (b) These molecules bind to their specific receptors located on the cell membrane, and induce growth and cell division of prostatic epithelium and stroma

division, but is also involved in inducing programmed cell death by apoptosis (Figure 21).

Apoptosis in the prostate occurs in its most florid form after castration. Within hours of withdrawal of androgen support to the epithelium of the prostate, nuclear condensation begins to develop as a result of the production of a number of endonucleases, which act to cleave the genomic DNA. A number of so-called apoptosis genes are involved in this process, including the *bcl*-2 gene and the *bax* gene. The visible result is condensation of the nucleus into so-called apoptotic bodies; these fragment and are eventually phagocytosed by macrophages, thereby permitting the breakdown products of intracellular structures to be reutilized.

Several of the molecular mechanisms by which cell-to-cell signalling by growth factor (cytokine) proteins is accomplished have recently been elucidated. Binding of growth factor signal molecules to the external component of the receptor appears to induce a conformational change in the intracellular component. Such a change results in the activation of tyrosine kinase, by the donation of a high-energy phosphate molecule as a result of conversion of guanine triphosphate (GTP) to guanine diphosphate (GDP). This process results in amplification of the signal within the cell; this, in turn, stimulates both cell growth and initiates mitosis (Figure 22).

Factors such as the fos and jun proteins, encoded by the c-*fos* and c-*jun* proto-oncogenes, are intimately concerned with growth regulation. Their intracellular production is enhanced by growth stimulatory factors such as EGF. The fos and jun proteins bind to specific recognition sites on the genome, characterized by the nucleotide sequence TGACTCA (Figure 23). This recognition site is

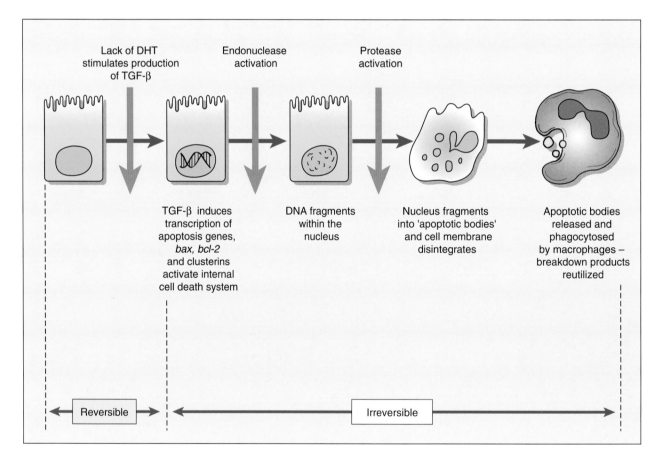

Figure 21 Apoptosis, or programmed cell death, is the normal mechanism by which homeostasis in the prostate is maintained. Apoptosis inducers, such as transforming growth factor-β (TGF-β), trigger the transcription of specific genes, such as *bax* and *bcl*-2, which influence the transcription of a number of endonucleases. These fragment the DNA within the nucleus and result in the formation of endonuclear apoptotic bodies. Subsequently, the cell itself disintegrates, and its constituents are engulfed by macrophages and reutilized for new cell formation

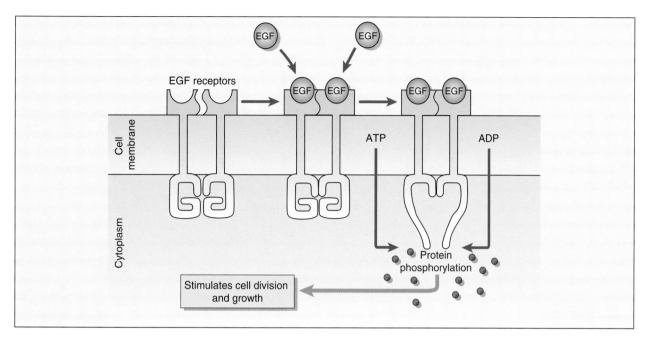

Figure 22   Growth factors such as epidermal growth factor (EGF) act as signal molecules on specific receptors on the cell membrane. The binding of EGF to its receptor results in a number of intracellular changes that culminate in cell growth and division

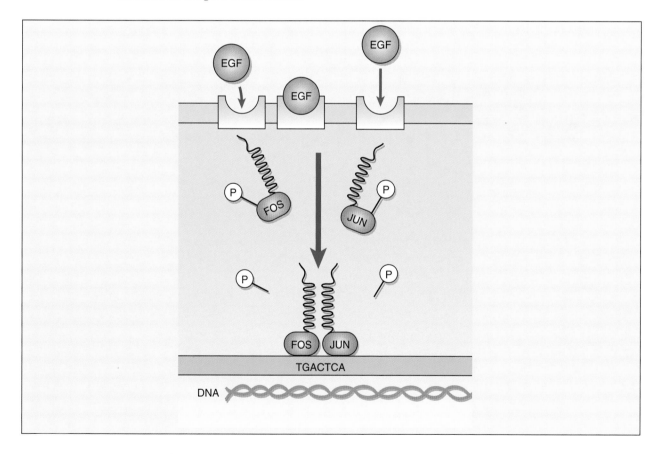

Figure 23   Factors such as the fos and jun proteins, encoded by the c-*fos* and c-*jun* proto-oncogenes, are intimately concerned with growth regulation. The fos and jun proteins bind as heterodimers to specific recognition sites on the genome, characterized by the nucleotide sequence TGACTCA which is adjacent to the androgen response element

closely associated with the androgen response area on the genome. This association allows 'cross-talk' between the two signalling pathways (Figure 24). Other pathways involved in prostate growth include the endothelin axis (Figure 25). Endothelin-1 (ET-1) induces cell proliferation by production of kinases involved in cell cycle regulation, including mitogen-activated protein kinase (MAPK), and inhibition of cell death (apoptosis).

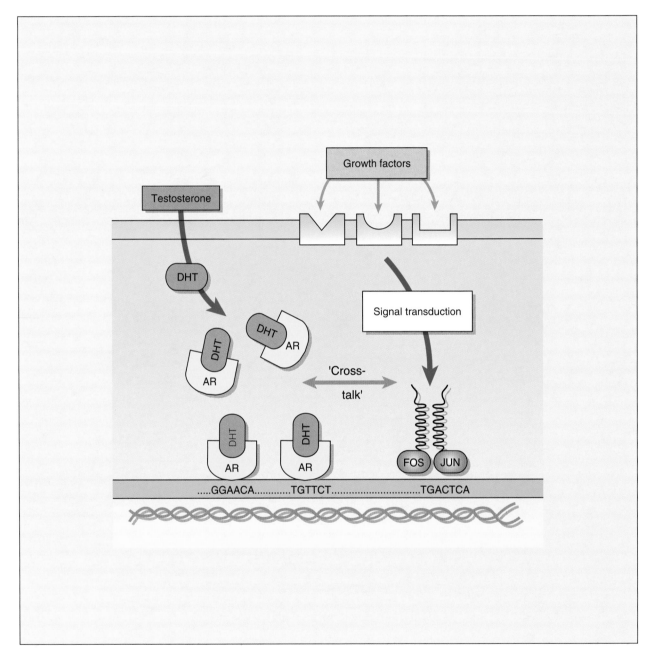

Figure 24   The proximity of the recognition sites to which the fos and jun proteins bind to the androgen response element allows 'cross-talk' between the two signalling pathways. It has been suggested that the association of DHT and the AR results in opening up of the DNA strands so as to provide better access for the transcription factors, thereby facilitating a more effective binding of the fos–jun heterodimer complex

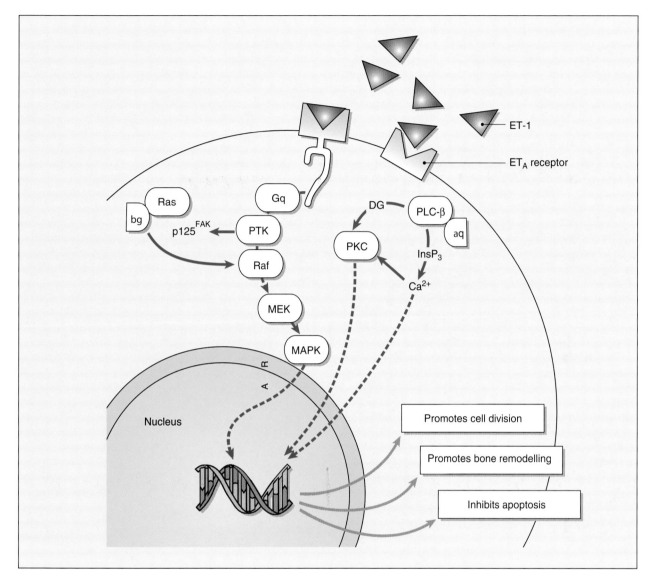

Figure 25 Stimulating the ET_A receptor with ET-1 triggers a signal transduction pathway that acts on a G protein (Gq) causing hydrolysis of phospholipase-C (PLC-β) and forming diacylglycerol (DG) and inositol 1,4,5 triphosphate ($InsP_3$). Intracellular calcium is mobilized from cytoplasmic stores by $InsP_3$, and, acting with DG, activates protein kinase C (PKC) and subsequently the Raf/MEK/MAPK pathway. Activated MAPK (mitogen-activated protein kinase) induces the transcription of the proto-oncogenes c-*fos*, c-*myc* and c-*jun*, resulting in cell growth and proliferation

6

Adrenoceptor signal transduction

The neurotransmitter molecule norepinephrine (noradrenaline) is located within dense-core vesicles in sympathetic nerve terminals located within the prostate. The arrival of nerve impulses at the nerve endings provokes norepinephrine release by a process of fusion of these vesicles with the cell membrane of the nerve endings. Norepinephrine then diffuses across the synaptic gap to activate either α_1-adrenoceptors, situated on the membrane of prostatic smooth muscle cells, or α_2-adrenoceptors, located on the nerve terminal itself (Figure 26). These α_2-adrenoceptors are autoregulatory in function and their blockade, by non-specific α-adrenoceptor blockers such as phenoxybenzamine, results in raised circulatory catecholamine levels with a consequent induction of tachycardia and palpitations.

The α_1-adrenoceptors located on the smooth muscle cell membrane are now known to consist of seven transmembrane domains and are linked intracellularly to a guanidine nucleotide binding protein (G protein) mechanism. Signal transduction results in G protein-linked activation of phospholipase C and the donation of a high-energy phosphate molecule from GTP. Signal amplification is accomplished by a molecular cascade, involving phosphotidylinositol and inositol triphosphate, which results in an influx of intracellular calcium, producing smooth muscle contractions as well as activation of protein kinase C, which, in turn, induces other intracellular metabolic responses[13] (Figure 27).

It has now been established that there are three subtypes of α_1-adrenoceptor (Figure 28). These have been cloned[14] and termed α_{1A}, α_{1B} and α_{1D}. The α_{1A} subtype appears to subserve mainly prostatic smooth muscle contraction; in contrast, the α_{1B} variety is involved in the maintenance of vasoconstrictor tone. α_{1D} Receptors are present in the detrusor muscle itself.

Recently, a fourth isoform of the receptor has been reported, but not yet cloned, which has a low affinity for prazosin, the original α_1-selective adrenoceptor blocker; the isoform has been dubbed the α_{1L} subtype. This discovery has laid a path towards the development of α-adrenoceptor blockers that are selective for one specific subtype – in other words, a 'prostate-selective' α-blocker – which may still be efficacious on the prostate, but with less effect on the cardiovascular system.

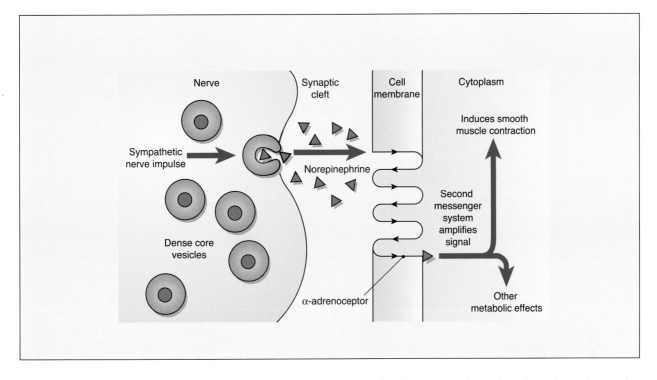

Figure 26   Norepinephrine acts as the main signal molecule at the adrenoceptor located on the cell membrane of prostatic smooth muscle cell. Norepinephrine is stored in dense-core vesicles within sympathetic nerve terminals. The arrival of an impulse at the nerve ending stimulates the release of norepinephrine, which then diffuses across the synaptic gap to interact with postsynaptic adrenoceptors, mainly of the α_1 subtype

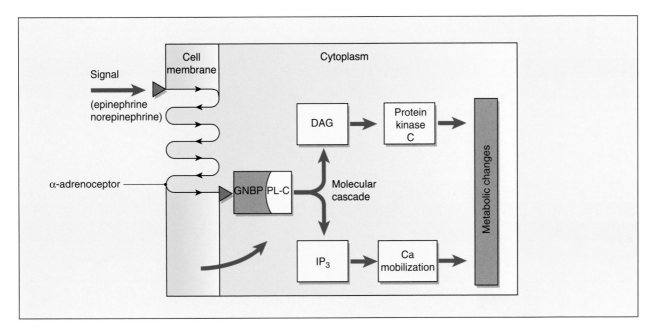

Figure 27   Signal transduction at the adrenoceptor is coupled to guanidine nucleotide binding protein (GNBP), the so-called G protein. Amplification of the signal involves both phosphotidylinositol and inositol triphosphate (IP_3), and induces a molecular cascade that results in smooth muscle relaxation and a number of longer-term metabolic responses, including the induction of both smooth muscle hypertrophy and hyperplasia

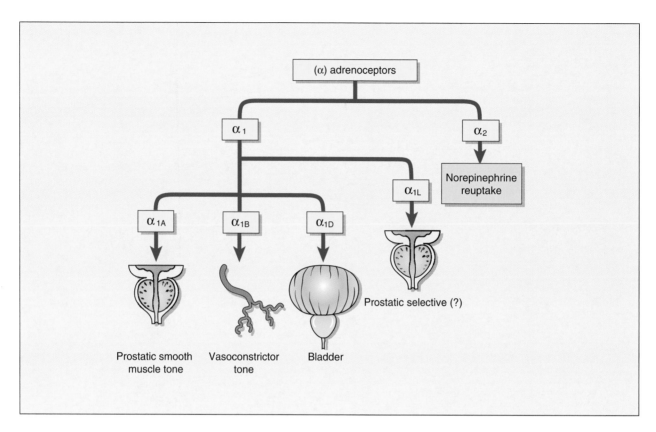

Figure 28   Originally subdivided into α_1- and α_2-adrenoceptors, a number of subtypes of the α_1-adrenoceptor have recently been identified and denoted α_{1A}, α_{1B} and α_{1D}. A fourth subtype, which has a low affinity for prazosin, has been dubbed the α_{1L} receptor. It is believed that the α_{1A} receptor mainly subserves prostatic smooth muscle contraction, whereas the α_{1B} receptor subtype is principally involved in control of vasoconstrictor tone. The α_{1L} receptor may also be responsible for some element of prostatic smooth muscle contraction

7

Causes of abnormal prostate cell growth

Two of the three dominant pathologies affecting the prostate gland, namely, benign prostatic hyperplasia and prostate cancer, are characterized by excessive cell proliferation. In contrast, prostatitis is predominantly an inflammatory disorder. In benign prostatic hyperplasia, the benign proliferative process affects both epithelial and stromal cells of the transitional zone. In contrast, prostate cancer is found more commonly in the peripheral zone, where it arises from atypical luminal cells or their stem cells.

Abnormal cell growth and division in the prostate may, in part, be the result of activation of oncogenes. Several of these have been implicated in the pathogenesis of prostate cancer, and it is plausible that they may also underlie the benign proliferative process of benign prostatic hyperplasia.

ONCOGENES

The *ras* proto-oncogene is normally involved in the regulation of cell growth and division. A mutation (Figure 29), resulting in a single base-pair change, causes an inability to separate GTP from the *ras* p21 protein, thereby locking it permanently in its activated form. The result is a continuing inappropriate signal for cell proliferation (Figure 30).

Another oncogene, c-*erb* B-2, acts through a different mechanism. A point mutation of DNA segment coding for c-*erb* B-2 results in the production of a distorted version of the EGF receptor. This mutant protein has no external component, with the result that the internal component continually signals the need for cell division, regardless of the presence or absence of EGF signal molecules[15] (Figure 31).

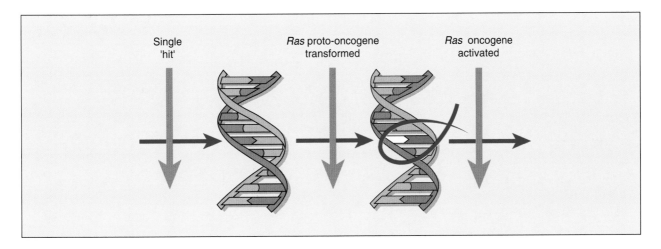

Figure 29   Oncogenesis within the prostate is due to the conversion of proto-oncogenes to active oncogenes. In the case of the *ras* oncogene, this occurs as a result of a mutation, or 'hit', involving alteration of a single nucleotide base-pair

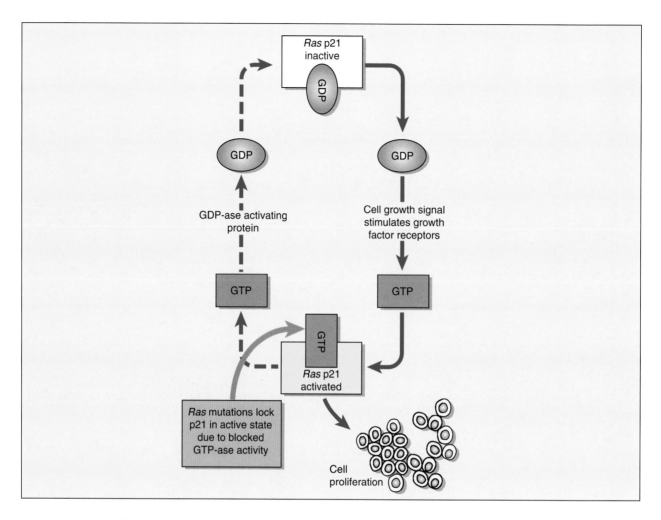

Figure 30   The mutated *ras* oncogene p21 protein cannot be deactivated by guanosine triphosphate (GTP) cyclase and thus continues to signal inappropriately for cell growth and division

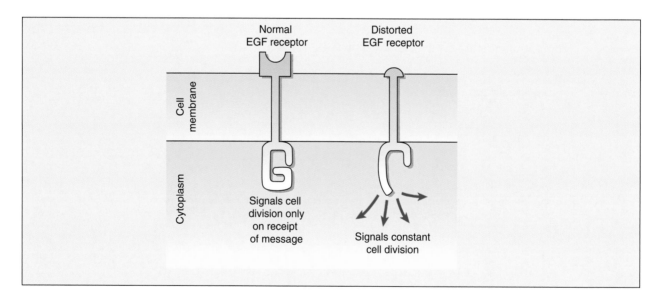

Figure 31   c-*erb* B-2 oncogene activation involves the production of truncated versions of the EGF receptor. The truncated receptor signals for continued cell growth and division, regardless of the presence or absence of EGF signal molecules

TUMOR SUPPRESSOR GENES

As well as the influence of growth-promoting onco-genes, abnormal prostate cell growth may also be the result of loss of the growth-restraining influences of one or more tumor suppressor genes[16], the best examples of which are the p53 and retinoblastoma tumor suppressor genes[17,18]. The p53 protein encoded by the former gene acts as an important regulator of cell division. Point mutation or complete deletion of this gene permits abnormal cell proliferation to occur (Figure 32).

The p53 tumor suppressor gene has also been implicated as an important factor in the development of other cancers, including lung, breast, colon and bladder neoplasms[19,20].

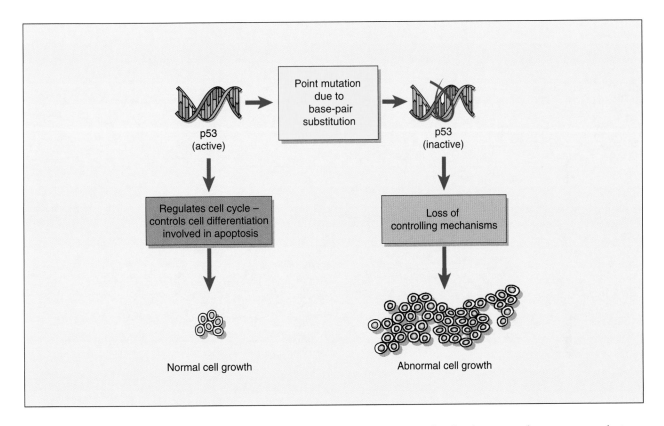

Figure 32   Tumor suppressor genes such as p53 are also important in the development of prostatic neoplasia. Normally, the p53 protein is involved in the regulation of cell division. Mutation or deletion of the gene thus encourages uncontrolled cell division

8

Local growth potential versus metastatic capacity

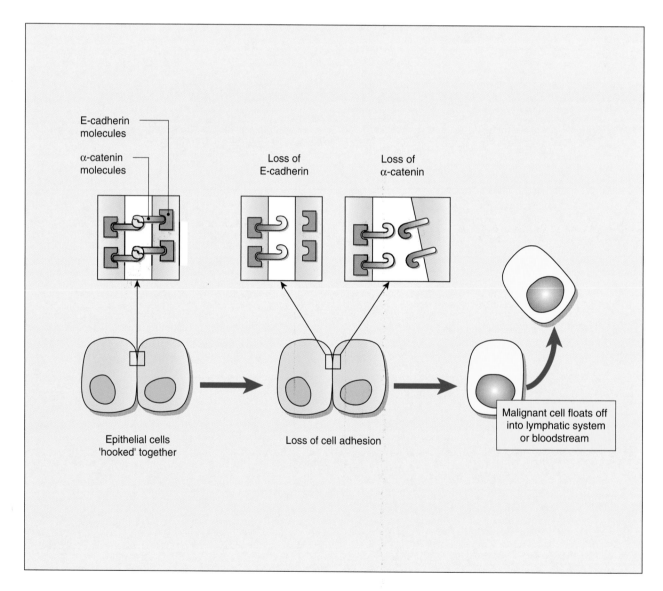

Figure 33   Local cell proliferation and metastatic capacity are different entities. Critical to the development of metastases is the loss of cell adhesion molecules such as E-cadherin. Absence of E-cadherin allows prostate cancer cells to 'float off' into the circulation and promotes the development of metastases. In the case of prostate cancer, these most frequently occur in bone or lymphatic tissues

Mutation or deletion of either proto-oncogenes or tumor suppressor genes may confer the potential for uncontrolled cell division and local growth but, for metastasis to occur, several further mutations are probably necessary.

In the normal prostate, epithelial cells are tightly bound to one another by cell adhesion molecules, such as E-cadherin, which is linked intracellularly to α-catenin. Deletion of the gene encoding either of these important proteins may facilitate the metastatic process by allowing malignant cells to migrate into the lymphatics and bloodstream (Figure 33). Loss of E-cadherin-staining in prostate cancer specimens appears to be strongly correlated with the subsequent development of metastases and is associated with a poor prognosis in prostate cancer patients.

ANGIOGENESIS FACTORS

For prostate cancer metastases to develop, tumor cells not only have to be released into lymphatics or the blood circulation, but cells must also have the ability to implant elsewhere and grow. Critical to this process is the ability of the developing metastases to induce their own blood supply – a process termed angiogenesis (Figure 34). This process depends on a number of proteins known collectively as angiogenesis factors, which appear to be important in conferring metastatic potential[21,22]. Prostate cancer has a particular proclivity for metastasis to bone. Many tumor-associated factors can stimulate osteoblastic metastases (Figure 35). These include insulin-like growth factors (IGF-1 and IGF-2), transforming growth factors (TGF-β), fibroblast growth factors (FGF-1 and FGF-2), bone morphogenes (BMPs), platelet-derived growth factors (PdGF) and endothelin-1 (ET-1). ET-1-induced angiogenesis further promotes osteoblastic metastases from the primary tumor.

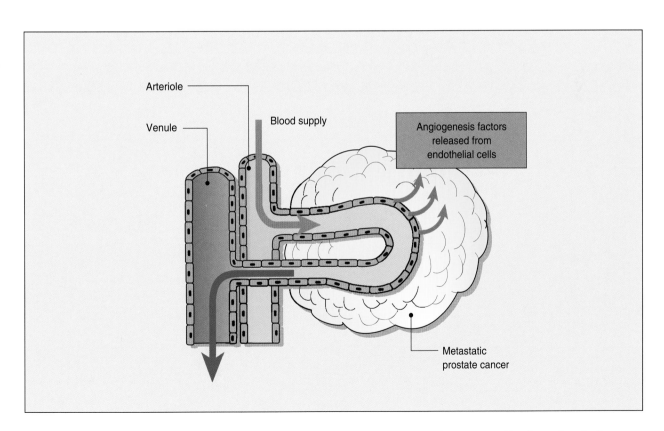

Figure 34 Angiogenesis describes the ability of a metastatic deposit to induce its own blood supply, which may be critical to its survival. A number of so-called angiogenesis factors have been implicated in metastatic prostate cancer

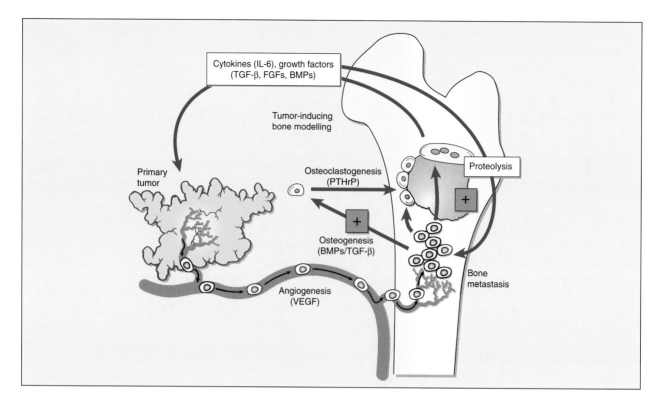

Figure 35 Many tumor-associated factors can directly stimulate osteoblastic metastases including insulin-like growth factors (IGF-1 and IGF-2), transforming growth factor (TGF-β), fibroblast growth factors (FGF-1 and PGF-2), platelet derived growth factors (PdGF) and endothelin-1 (ET-1). PSA and urokinase-type activator (uPA) act indirectly by activating latent TGF-β and reducing the inhibitory binding proteins such as IGF-binding proteins. ET-1-induced angiogenesis further promotes osteoblastic metastases from the primary tumor

9

Stepwise induction of prostatic neoplasia

Neoplastic change in prostatic cells is not simply the result of a single mutational event, but rather a series of sequential interrelated mutations. The precise sequence of these events in prostatic neoplasia has yet to be elucidated, but a putative molecular scenario is depicted in Figure 36.

Activation of the *ras* and c-*erb* B-2 oncogenes, and deletion of the p53 tumor suppressor gene, may occur in a stepwise fashion. These changes confer local growth potential on prostatic epithelium, but metastatic capacity awaits further mutations involving deletions of cell adhesion molecules such as E-cadherin and the ability to elaborate angiogenesis factors.

The considerable time required for this sequential series of intracellular events to occur may account for the observation that prostate cancer very seldom develops in men below 40 years of age and usually presents clinically in men beyond middle age.

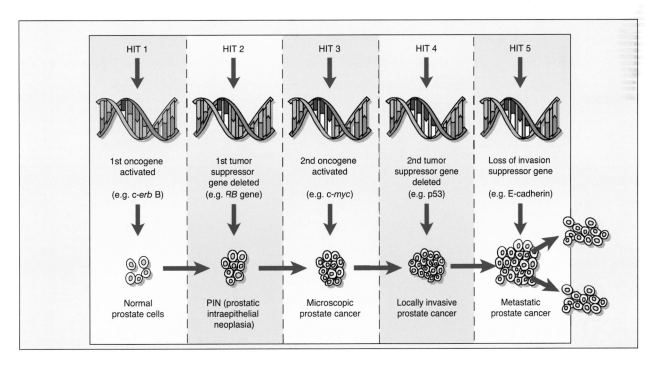

Figure 36 The development of prostate cancer is a multi-step process involving the activation of oncogenes, such as *ras* and c-*erb* B-2, and the loss of tumor suppressor genes, such as p53 and the retinoblastoma (RB) tumor suppressor gene. Metastatic capacity is then bestowed by the deletion of the cell adhesion molecule E-cadherin and the release of angiogenesis factors. A putative pathway of prostate carcinogenesis is illustrated here

10

Inflammatory processes and the prostate

For reasons not yet understood, the prostate seems especially prone to chronic inflammation. In approximately 10% of cases, this is the result of a bacterial, chlamydial or other infecting microorganism. For the remaining 90% of cases, however, no definite etiological cause has yet been identified.

Prostatic ducts, and the acini into which they branch (see Figure 5), are the foci of these inflammatory processes. A number of non-infective etiological factors may be involved. When inflammation does occur, the subsequent chronic prostatitis affects the peripheral zone more often than the central zone of the gland. One explanation for this may be that peripheral zone prostatic ducts enter the prostatic urethra at a less oblique angle than do central zone ducts. This may render the peripheral zone ducts more susceptible to intraprostatic reflux of urine during micturition (Figure 37).

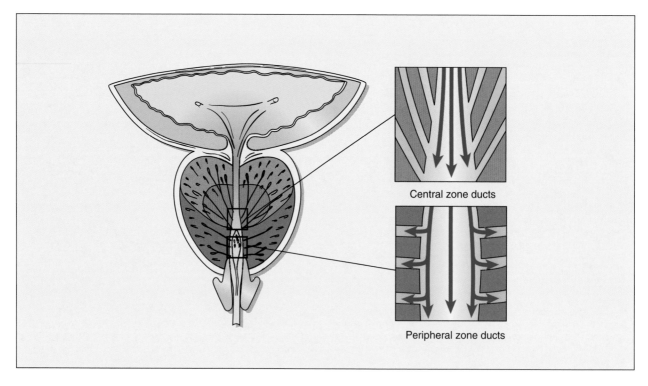

Central zone ducts

Peripheral zone ducts

Figure 37   Prostatitis is characterized by the development of chronic inflammation, especially involving the peripheral zone of the prostate. Intraprostatic reflux of urine into the horizontally situated peripheral zone ducts may be one of the triggering mechanisms involved

Studies using intravesical instillation of India ink prior to voiding and subsequent prostatectomy have revealed an intraprostatic finding of carbon particles (Figure 38) and have also demonstrated their subsequent ingestion by macrophages[23] (Figure 39).

Urine reflux into prostatic ducts (Figure 40) may not only be one mechanism of induction of chronic inflammation, but may also be the cause of intra-prostatic calculus formation (Figure 41). Studies have revealed that, whereas many prostatic calculi

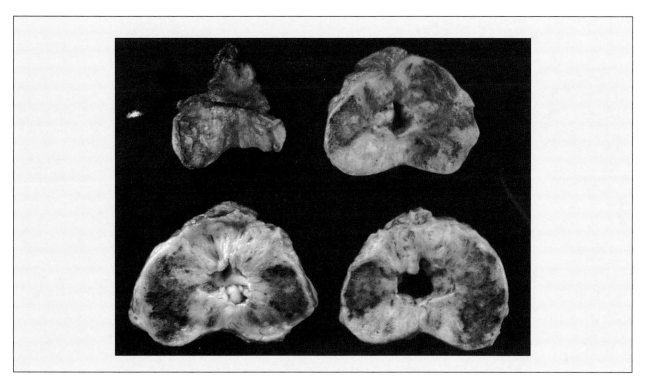

Figure 38   Carbon particles (India ink) placed in the bladder and subsequently voided could be demonstrated in the prostatic ducts of patients who subsequently underwent prostatectomy

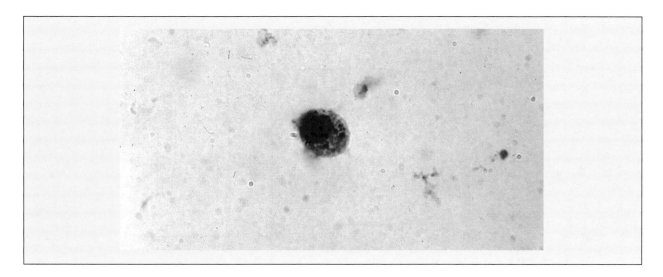

Figure 39   Fluid expressed from the prostatic ducts several days after placement of India ink in the bladder shows ingestion of carbon particles by macrophages, thus confirming the presence of intraprostatic reflux in a patient with prostatitis

are formed as a result of concretions of prostatic gland secretions, many are composed of similar constituents to those of renal, ureteric and bladder calculi (urinary constituents), thereby confirming the tendency of urine to enter the prostate.

Whatever the cause of the inflammatory process of prostatitis, once initiated, the disorder tends to become chronic in nature. Activation of complement and the involvement of macrophages are both central to this on-going inflammatory process (Figure 42).

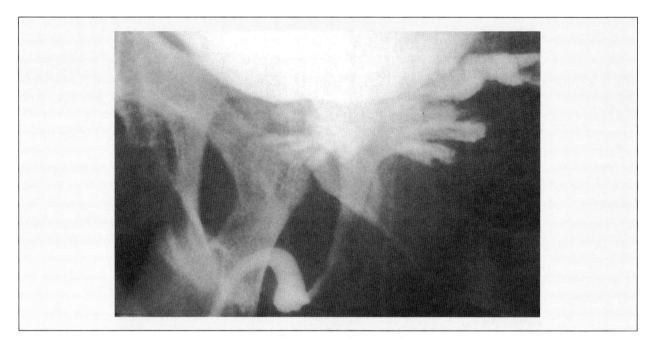

Figure 40   Intraprostatic reflux can be demonstrated during the performance of a voiding cystourethrogram

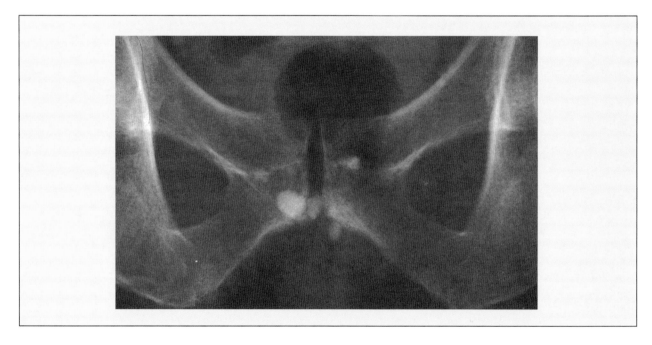

Figure 41   Prostatic calculi can be seen on a plain X-ray, perhaps secondary to intraprostatic urinary reflux. Calculi tend to form within the prostate, where they may constitute a nidus for chronic prostatic infection

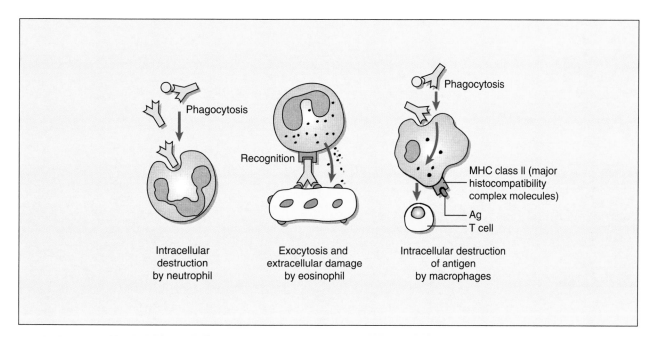

Figure 42 Prostatitis is characterized by an inflammatory response within the gland. Neutrophils and macrophages phagocytose and destroy antigens such as those presented by bacterial cell walls intracellularly. However, macrophages and other cells of this lineage also present antigen. In contrast, eosinophil killing is guided by antibody and receptor interaction, and effected extracellularly

11

Pathology of the prostate

Accurate histological identification of the three basic pathological processes that affect the prostate – adenocarcinoma, benign prostatic hyperplasia and prostatitis – is central to accurate diagnosis and correct institution of therapy. Whereas a detailed exposition of the many less commonly encountered variations of prostatic pathology is beyond the scope of this Atlas, the classical appearances of the most prevalent disorders are described and illustrated here.

BENIGN PROSTATIC HYPERPLASIA

Histological benign prostatic hyperplasia is classically characterized by a mixed proliferation of both stromal and epithelial elements to form nodules (Figures 43 and 44). There are, however, individual variations, with some patients developing a predominantly stromal version of the disease and others showing mainly epithelial overgrowth (Figure 45).

The luminal-to-basal cell relationship is retained in epithelial hyperplasia, which is not considered to be a premalignant condition. Subgroups of epithelial hyperplasia include basal cell (Figure 46) and cribriform hyperplasia. However, their only importance is the occasional difficulty in distinguishing them from cancer.

PROSTATE CANCER

There is now evidence to suggest that many prostate cancers are preceded or accompanied by a pre-malignant change in the luminal cells, known as prostatic intraepithelial neoplasia (PIN)[24]. The condition is characterized by progressive dysplasia of the prostatic epithelium, initially within an intact basal cell layer. PIN was initially subdivided into mild, moderate and severe forms[25], but the terms 'low-grade' and 'high-grade' are now preferred[26] (Figures 47 and 48).

Essential for the diagnosis of actual prostate carcinoma rather than pre-malignant PIN is the demonstration of invasion: carcinoma lacks basal cells, whereas PIN may have an intact or intermittent basal cell layer. This difference reflects the tendency of neoplastic prostatic epithelial cells to invade the

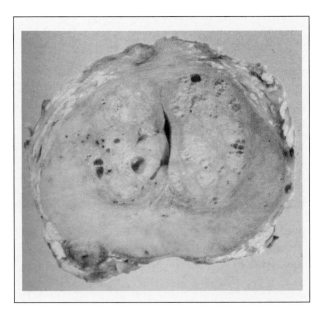

Figure 43   Transverse section of a prostate (5 cm across) showing bilateral hyperplastic nodules which have reduced the urethra to a slit. In contrast, the carcinoma is seen as solid homogeneous tissue posteriorly (on the left extending to the right)

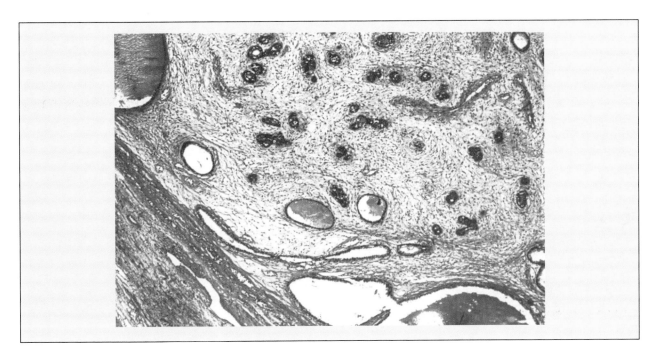

Figure 44   Hyperplastic nodules, composed of epithelium and stroma, can be seen here compressing the adjacent gland (H & E)

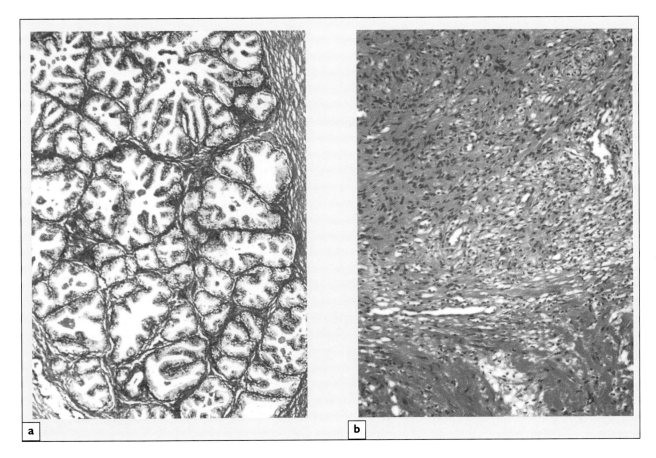

Figure 45   Hyperplastic nodules may be due to either predominantly epithelial (a) or stromal (b) overgrowth. Stromal nodules are almost always periurethral and are often situated immediately beneath the urethral epithelium (H & E)

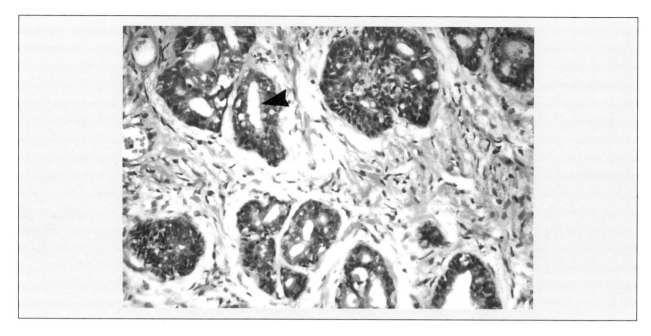

Figure 46   Basal cell hyperplasia: the basal cells have produced a stratified layer that has compressed the tall columnar cells into a narrow rim. These small hyperchromatic acini may be misdiagnosed as cancer, but the double-cell layer (comprising LP34-positive outer basal cells and compressed PSA-positive luminal cells) confirms the benign nature of this appearance (H & E)

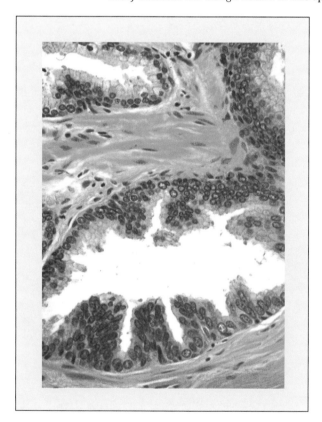

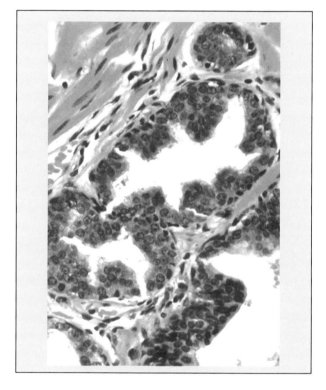

Figure 48   High-grade prostatic intraepithelial neoplasia: the luminal epithelium is stratified, but the cells have lost their polarity. The nuclei are larger than normal and contain nucleoli. In this section, an outer layer of basal cells can still be seen (H & E)

Figure 47   Low-grade prostatic intraepithelial neoplasia (lower field): the luminal epithelium is stratified and the nuclei are larger than that of the normal acinus (upper field) (H & E)

basement membrane. Identification of this process of invasion can be facilitated by the use of immunocytochemistry to delineate basal cells and the cytokeratin of the basement membrane (Figure 49; *see also* Figure 6).

Once invasion has occurred, the histological grading of the malignancy is accomplished by use of

Gleason's technique[27], which is based on the tendency of a given tumor to form gland-like structures (Figure 50). Because of the marked heterogeneity of prostatic cancers, the Gleason score is calculated as the sum of the two most dominant histological patterns within a given cancer.

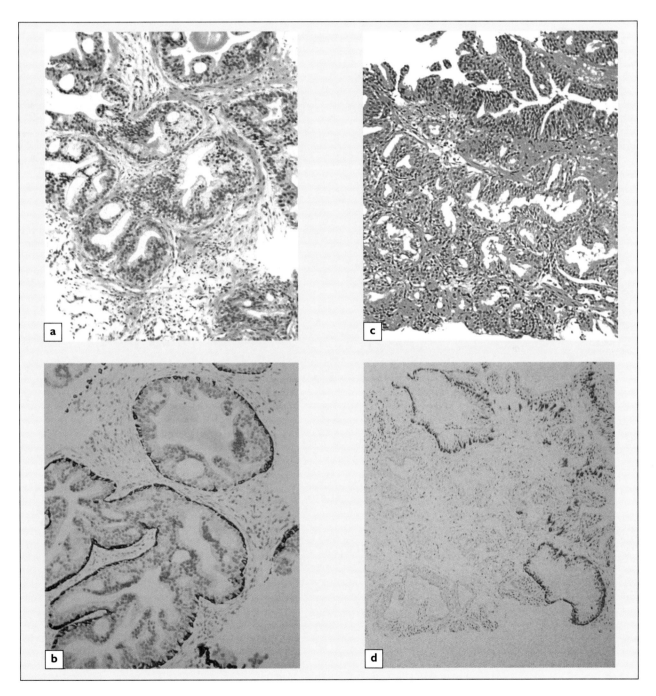

Figure 49 Prostatic intraepithelial neoplasia compared with carcinoma: prostatic intraepithelial neoplasia may resemble cancer architecturally and/or cytologically (a) with H & E staining, but can be shown to have a basal cell layer (b) immunocytochemically whereas, with carcinoma (c), the basal cell layer cannot be demonstrated (d); the positive staining is found only in residual benign ducts or acini

Gleason scores 2–4 are well differentiated (Figures 51 and 52), scores 5–7 are moderately well differentiated (Figures 53 and 54) and scores 8–10 are poorly differentiated varieties of prostate adenocarcinoma. These tumor gradings appear to correlate well with subsequent metastatic potential and overall survival. Cancers originating in the transitional zone tend to have a lower Gleason grade than tumors of the peripheral zone, an observation that appears to correlate well with the higher proliferative rates seen in the latter (Figure 55).

Further information concerning the biological aggressiveness of the cancer can be gleaned from features such as perineural invasion (Figure 56), infiltration of the capsule, adjacent adipose tissue or striated muscle, as well as seminal vesicle invasion (Figure 57). A number of new techniques which show promise in terms of prediction of subsequent tumor behavior include the assessment of the

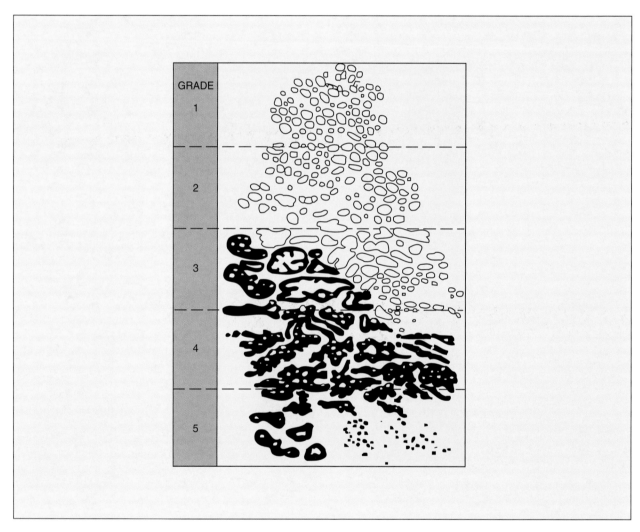

Figure 50 The Gleason grading system is the most widely used system for grading prostatic adenocarcinoma. Devised during the Veterans Administration Cooperative Urological Research Group studies (1960–1975), different tumor patterns were identified without preconceived rating. Their presence was recorded and subsequently correlated with survival data by the study statistician. The patterns were arranged into five grades, numbered in order of increasing malignancy as determined by the mortality data. The methodology has stood the test of time. As prostatic adenocarcinoma is morphologically heterogeneous and does not appear to be 'as bad as its worst part', but behaves in accordance with its average morphology, the two dominant grades are identified and summated to arrive at a Gleason score (for example, grade 3 + grade 2 = Gleason score 5) for a given patient

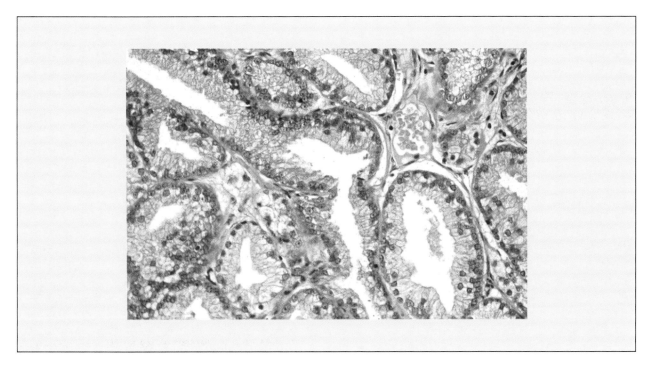

Figure 51   Gleason grade 2: this is characterized by closely packed acini. Gleason grade 1 is similar, but has acini which are more constant in size and form nodules with a well-defined edge. Gleason grades 1 and 2 are most frequently diagnosed in biopsy specimens

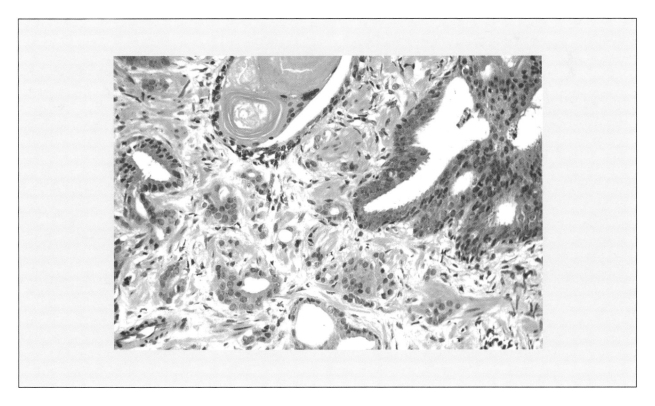

Figure 52   Gleason grade 3: these are typically small, angular, malignant acini that form an irregular mass and infiltrate benign acini at the edge of the lesion. In this section, there is a benign acinus containing corpora amylacea (top of field); prostatic intraepithelial neoplasia is also present (on the right)

tendency of the tumor to form new blood vessels (neovascularity)[28], or stain for anti-cathepsin β or stefin A[29].

HISTOLOGY OF PROSTATE METASTASES

Most prostate cancer metastases are readily identifiable as being consistent with the previously diagnosed prostatic primary. However, in those patients in whom metastases are the presenting feature, or where the secondary deposit is poorly differentiated, then immunocytochemical detection of PSA expression may be helpful (Figure 58).

HISTOLOGY OF PROSTATITIS

Histologically, prostatitis occurs in two major forms: acute – sometimes with abscess formation (Figure 59) – and chronic. Chronic prostatitis may be bacterial or abacterial, but histological examination cannot distinguish between the two (Figure 60). Atrophy is a common sequel (Figure 61). Granulomatous prostatitis may also occur (Figure 62), but tuberculous prostatitis is only occasionally seen nowadays. Intravesical BCG (*bacillus Calmette-Guérin*) vaccine therapy may, on occasions, result in a granulomatous prostatitis (Figure 63).

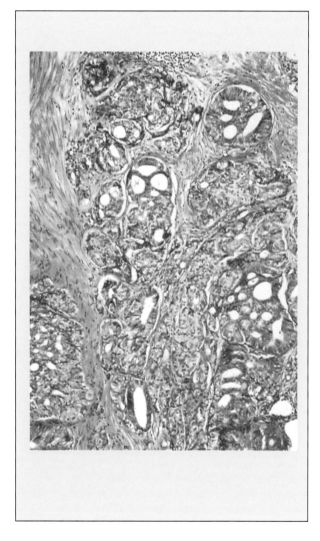

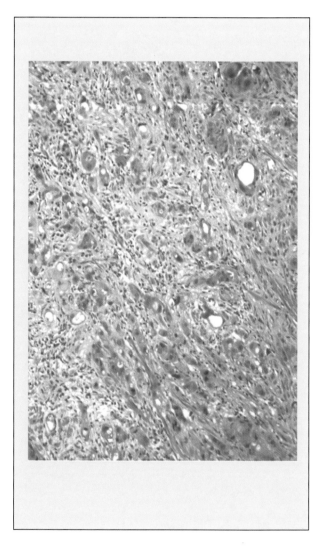

Figure 53   Gleason grade 4: the malignant acini fuse to form irregular masses, often with a cribriform result. A clear-celled 'hypernephroid' form is also described in this grading

Figure 54   Gleason grade 5: this is characterized by sheets of malignant cells with little evidence of gland formation. Single-celled infiltration is common

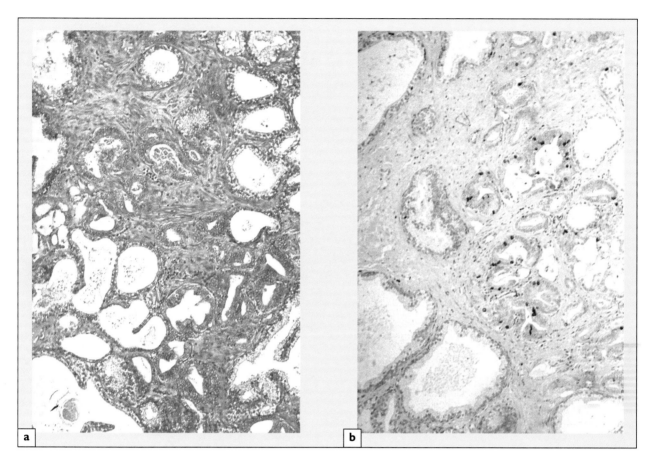

Figure 55   The proliferating fraction of the cells in adenocarcinoma is demonstrated by positive nuclear staining to antibody MIBI. With H & E (a), adenocarcinoma is seen towards the center of the field with peripheral benign acini. The contrast in proliferation fraction between these two areas is seen by immunocytochemical preparation (b)

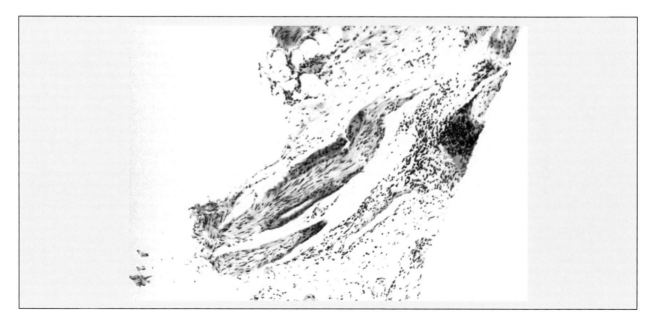

Figure 56   An adenocarcinoma is invading a nerve lying within adipose tissue at the edge of a biopsy core. The number and size of the nerves invaded by tumor correlate with the extraglandular extent of malignancy, as defined in radical prostatectomy specimens

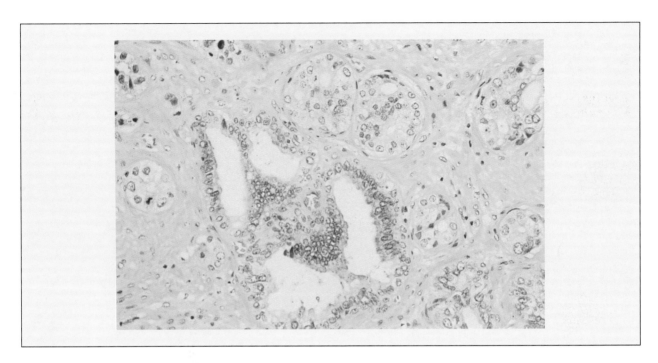

Figure 57   Adenocarcinoma can be seen spreading into a seminal vesicle. The benign, pigmented lining epithelium of the vesicle can be seen centrally

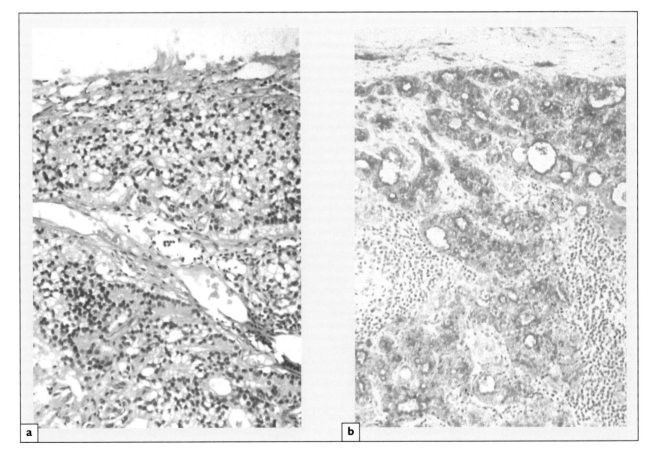

Figure 58   An adenocarcinoma can be seen infiltrating a lymph node from the obturator fossa with H & E staining (a) and with immunocytochemical preparation to demonstrate prostate-specific antigen (b)

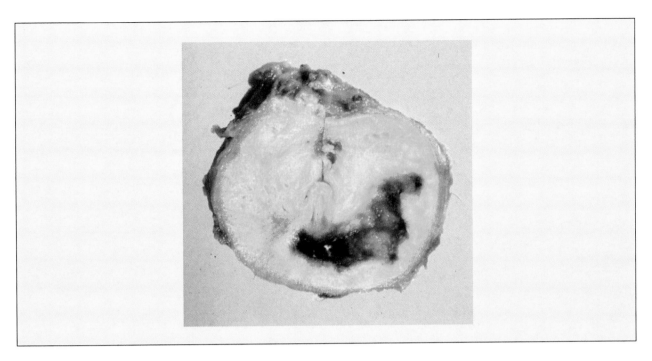

Figure 59   Transverse section of prostate showing a posteriorly situated abscess cavity on the left

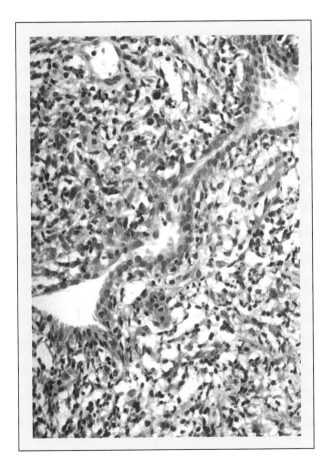

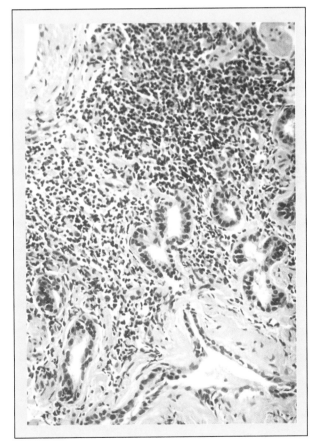

Figure 60   Prostatitis: an inflammatory infiltrate can be seen surrounding a duct or acinus and infiltrating the atrophic epithelium

Figure 61   Atrophy: a shrunken lobule is associated with the presence of fibrosis and chronic inflammatory cells

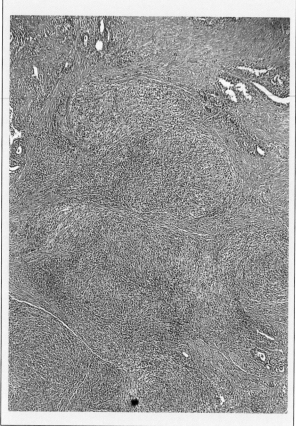

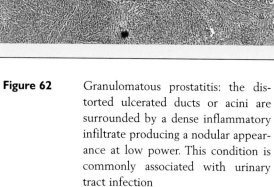

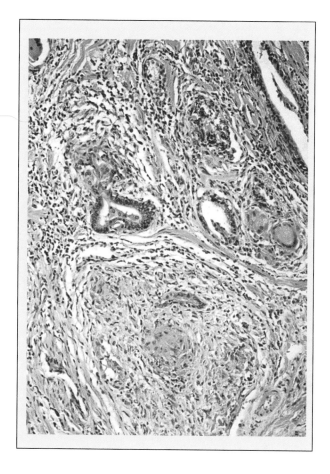

Figure 62 Granulomatous prostatitis: the distorted ulcerated ducts or acini are surrounded by a dense inflammatory infiltrate producing a nodular appearance at low power. This condition is commonly associated with urinary tract infection

Figure 63 Prostatitis after therapy with intravesical *bacillus Calmette-Guérin* (BCG) vaccine. The scattered well-defined granulomata contain Langhans' giant cells and occasional central caseation

12

Bladder outlet obstruction

Benign prostatic hyperplasia, prostate cancer and acute or chronic prostatitis may all result in bladder outlet obstruction. In addition, other non-prostatic disorders, such as bladder neck dyssynergia and urethral stricture disease (Figure 64), may also result in bladder outlet obstruction. In response to the changes associated with increased outflow resistance, the detrusor muscle undergoes hypertrophy, with the development of trabeculation. As a consequence

of these changes, lower urinary tract symptoms develop. The interrelationship between benign prostatic hyperplasia (prostatic enlargement), bladder outlet obstruction and lower urinary tract symptoms can be depicted in a Venn diagram (Figure 65). It should be recalled, however, that many factors other than benign prostatic hyperplasia can affect bladder function as men age (Figure 66).

Although bladder wall hypertrophy, which develops in response to the increased effort required

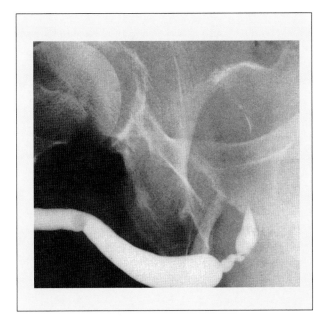

Figure 64 A retrograde urethrogram showing a stricture of the bulbar urethra. In older men, the bladder outflow obstruction resulting from such a stricture may mimic obstructive benign prostatic hyperplasia

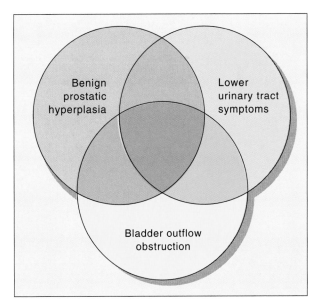

Figure 65 The three basic features of benign prostatic hyperplasia: hyperplasia (i.e. transitional zone enlargement with concomitant increase in overall gland volume), lower urinary tract symptoms, and bladder outflow obstruction

during voiding, is associated with an increase in size and strength of detrusor smooth muscle bundles, there is also infiltration by collagen (Figure 67) and a relative depletion of parasympathetic nerve endings. Thus, the overall efficiency of bladder contraction may be impaired, leading to the progressive development of post-void residual urine.

When bladder outlet obstruction is severe and bladder emptying is impaired, diverticular formation may develop, together with the formation of bladder calculi; only rarely these days do bilateral hydronephrosis and renal impairment occur (Figure 68).

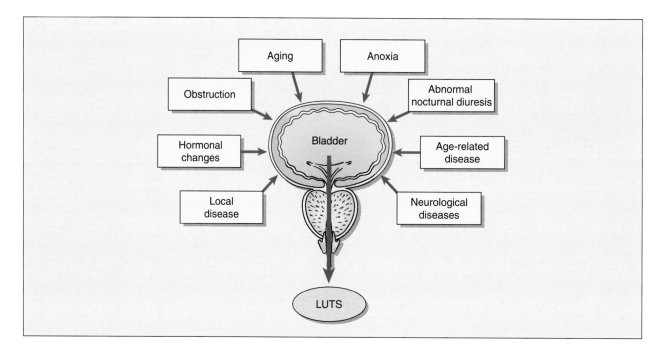

Figure 66 Although benign prostatic hyperplasia is the most common cause of lower urinary tract symptoms (LUTS), many other factors play a role

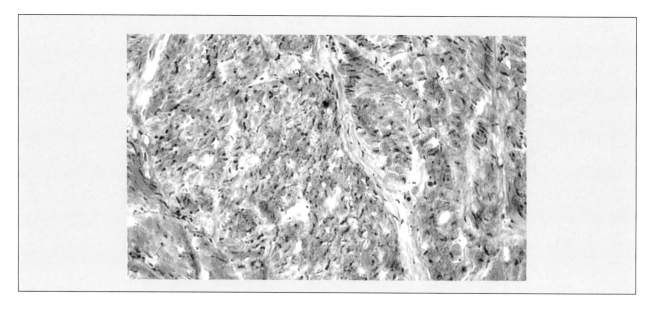

Figure 67 Collagen deposition has occurred between the smooth muscle cell bundles of the bladder detrusor muscle. This phenomenon is seen as part of the bladder response to the gradual development of obstruction (Masson trichrome)

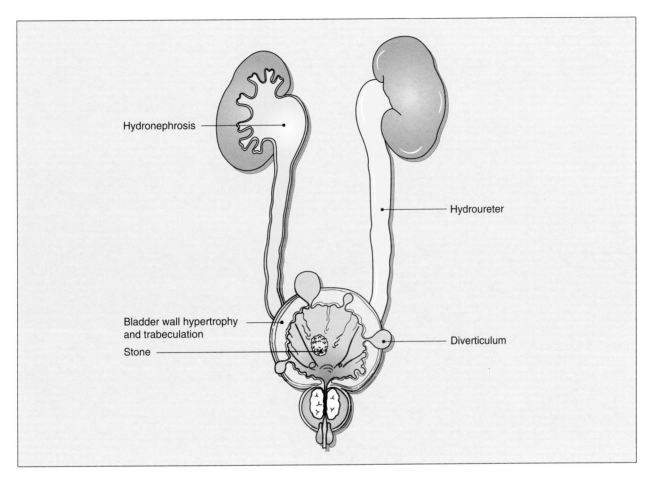

Figure 68   Secondary effects of obstructive benign prostatic hyperplasia include bladder wall hypertrophy with diverticula and bladder stone formation. The development of ureteric dilatation and bilateral hydronephrosis is less frequently seen

13

Progressive development of benign prostatic hyperplasia

As suggested by Berry and colleagues[30] on the basis of autopsy studies, benign prostatic hyperplasia is generally a gradually progressive disease that commences in men who are around 40 years of age (Figure 69). Data from the Baltimore Longitudinal Study of Aging[31] suggest that symptomatic benign prostatic hyperplasia also tends to progress with time in the majority of men (Figure 70). The average prostate volume increase is in the order of 0.6 ml per annum, and this is associated with a mean diminution of flow rate of 0.2 ml/s/year[32] (Figure 71). Recent data confirm that men with larger prostates and higher PSA values suffer a faster rate of disease progression than those with smaller glands (Figure 72)[33].

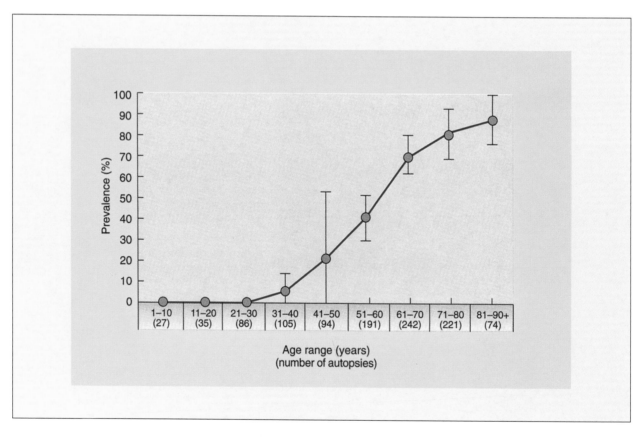

Figure 69   The prevalence of anatomical benign prostatic hyperplasia rises with age. By the age of 90 years, the disease is virtually universal in men (modified with permission from Berry et al.[30])

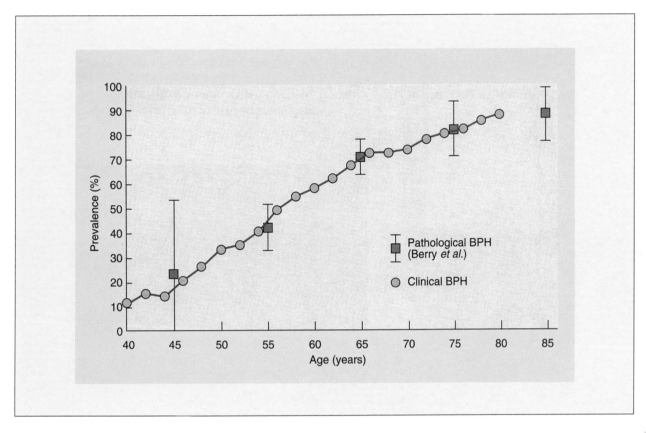

Figure 70 Data from the Baltimore Longitudinal Study of Aging suggest that the prevalence of symptomatic benign prostatic hyperplasia (BPH) also increases progressively with age (with permission from Arrighi et al.[31])

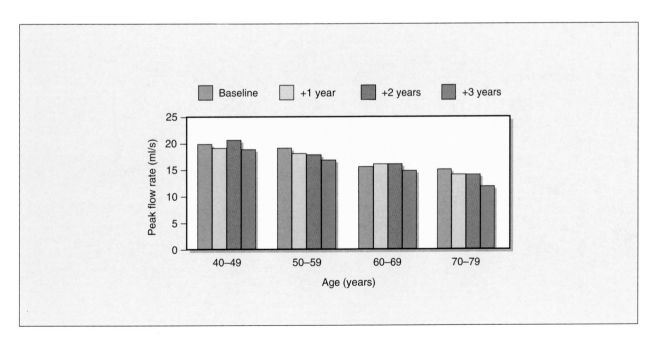

Figure 71 Decrease in maximum urinary flow rates over 3 years for different age groups detected in men from Olmstead County

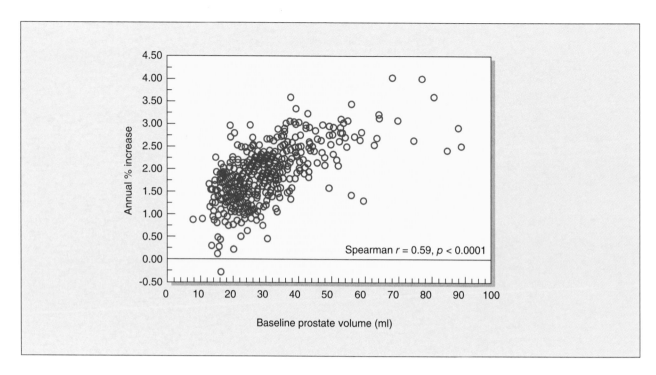

Figure 72   A plot of the baseline prostate volume against the annual percentage increase demonstrates that larger prostates grow more rapidly than smaller glands

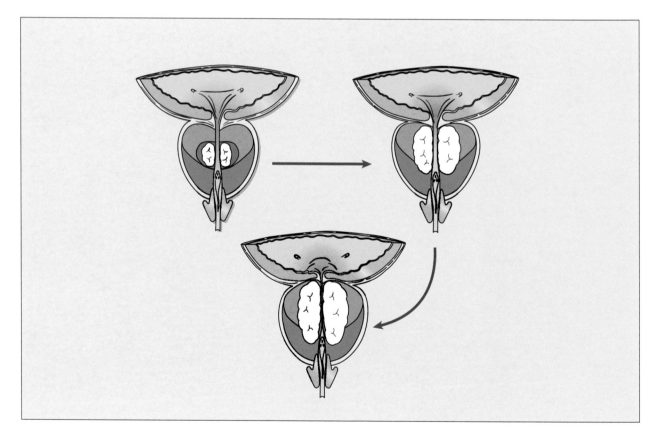

Figure 73   The progressive development of benign prostatic hyperplasia tissue in the transitional zone of the prostate often results in gradually increasing bladder outflow obstruction

The explanation for these findings lies in the progressive expansion of the transitional zone by the adenoma (Figure 73). This process reduces the distensibility of the urethra during voiding and produces gradually increasing bladder outlet obstruction. This increase in prostate volume is associated with a progressive risk of lower urinary tract symptoms, and a negative impact on quality of life. The increase in prostate volume is also associated with a rise in PSA value, which, in the absence of prostate cancer, can act as a useful surrogate for gland volume. Significantly, men with larger prostates and (since PSA provides a reflection of total prostate epithelial cell volume) higher PSA values are more likely to develop complications of benign prostatic hyperplasia such as acute urinary retention or require benign prostatic hyperplasia-related surgery (Figure 74). Other risk factors for acute urinary retention include severe symptoms and markedly reduced maximum urinary flow rates[34] (Figures 75 and 76).

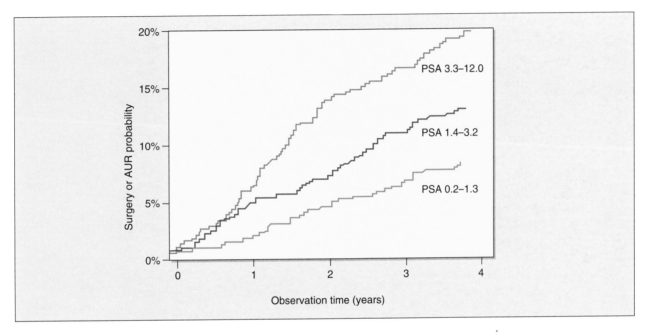

Figure 74   PSA values also act as a predictor of the need for benign prostatic hyperplasia-related surgery and the risk of acute urinary retention (AUR)

Olmstead County Community Observational Study (*n* = 2115) 8344 person-years of follow-up: 57 episodes AUR				
Incidence 6.8/1000 person-years				
Symptoms	40–49	50–59	60–69	70–79
None to mild	2.6	1.7	5.4	9.3
Moderate to severe	3.0	7.4	12.9	34.7
Risk increase 4-fold: flow rate < 12 ml/s 3-fold: prostate volume > 30 ml				

Figure 75   Risk factors for acute urinary retention (AUR) in the Olmstead County Study of 2115 men. Increase in severity of symptoms, reduced urinary flow rates and larger prostate volumes are all associated with an increased risk of acute urinary retention (modified with permission from Jacobsen *et al.*[34])

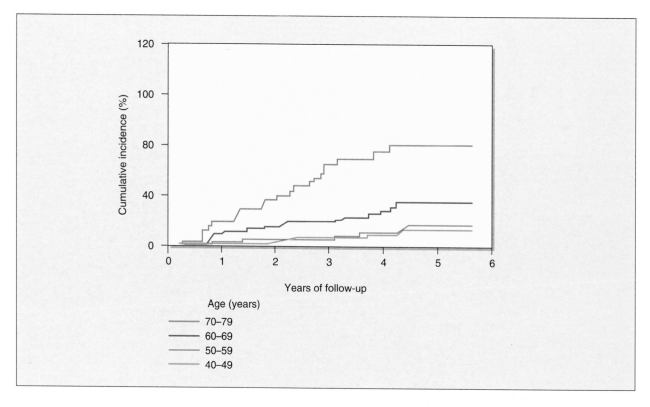

Figure 76   Cumulative incidence of acute urinary retention over 6 years. The risks of this complication of benign prostatic hyperplasia rise progressively with age

The anatomical distribution of the adenoma is not always uniform. When the process affects mainly the proximal periurethral zone, so-called median or middle lobe enlargement occurs (Figure 77). In this situation, the adenoma is often stromal rather than glandular in nature, is not detectable by digital rectal examination (DRE) and is commonly associated with a disproportionate amount of bladder outlet obstruction.

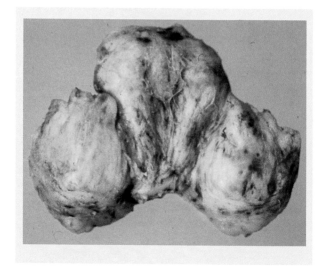

Figure 77   This resected prostate specimen shows enlargement of both so-called lateral lobes as well as of the middle lobe

14

Localized progression of prostate cancer

The majority of prostate cancers develop initially in the peripheral zone of the prostate, either from, or in conjunction with, prostatic epithelium neoplasia. They generally grow slowly at first, often with a cell-doubling time of more than 2 years. As dedifferentiation occurs due to sequential mutations, however, clonal selection results in an increase in the rate of cell division and the development of local invasion.

The TNM (tumors/nodes/metastases) staging system classifies prostate cancers locally as T1–4 (Figure 78). Impalpable tumors, which are now being detected with increasing frequency, are classified as T1A and T1B (according to grade and volume) when identified by transurethral resection (TUR; Figure 79), or as T1C if impalpable and detected purely on the basis of an elevated PSA and subsequent transrectal ultrasound (TRUS)-guided biopsy.

Local extension of prostate adenocarcinoma most frequently occurs through the prostatic capsule (so-called capsular extension) posterolaterally via perineural or lymphatic channels, which follow the prostatic branches of the neurovascular bundles of Walsh (Figures 80 and 81). For this reason, it is advised that, during a nerve-sparing radical retro-pubic prostatectomy, the neurovascular bundle on the affected side be sacrificed to reduce the chances of a positive margin in that location.

Further local extension most commonly involves the seminal vesicles, a pathological finding which is associated with a poor prognosis. Prostatic tumor may also directly infiltrate the bladder base and obstruct the ureteric orifices, producing hydro-nephrosis and, if bilateral, eventual anuria.

The ureters may also be obstructed by involved lymph nodes, usually at the level of the pelvic brim. Posterior extension of the tumor is less common, as Denonvilliers' fascia appears to act as an effective barrier to spread. Occasionally, however, prostate adenocarcinoma may encircle the rectum and obstruct the lower bowel (Figure 82).

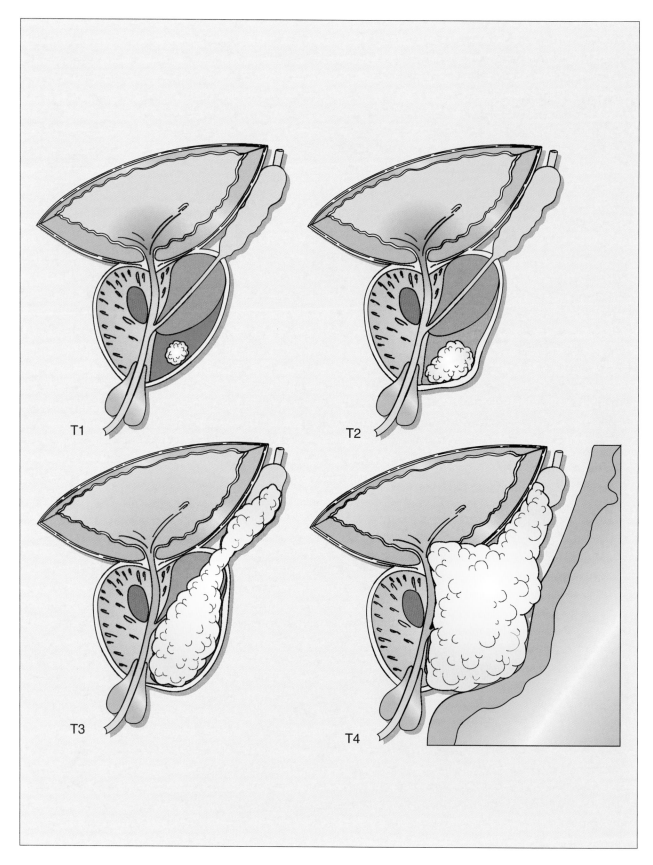

Figure 78   Clinical staging of prostate cancer: most prostate cancers develop in the peripheral zone and, when sufficiently large, become palpable as a T2 lesion. A T3 lesion denotes invasion of the prostatic capsule, and a T4 lesion often involves either the seminal vesicles or other adjacent structures

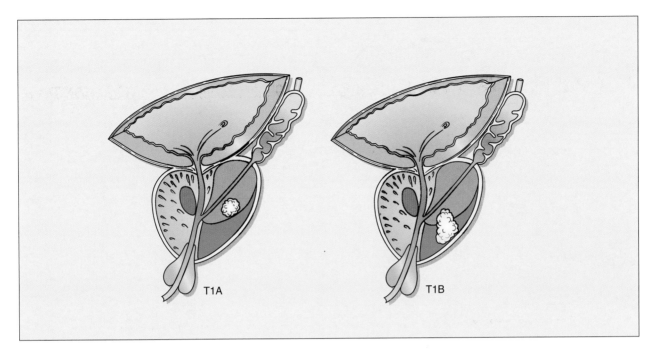

Figure 79   Impalpable prostate cancer is not infrequently diagnosed at the time of transurethral resection of the prostate (TURP). If the cancer is well differentiated and involves less than 5% of the resected material, it is classed as a T1A and carries a good prognosis. If, on the other hand, the lesion is moderately or poorly differentiated and involves more than 5% of the resected chippings, then it is termed a T1B lesion. These lesions are associated with a poorer prognosis and a higher probability that residual cancer will persist in the prostate remnant after resection and require further therapy

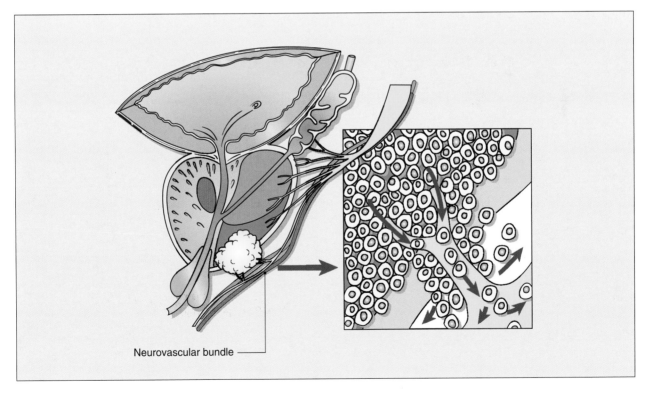

Figure 80   Because many prostate cancers develop posteriorly in the peripheral zone of the gland, it is not surprising that tumor cells are often able to escape the confines of the gland through the veins and lymphatics that accompany the neurovascular bundles of Walsh

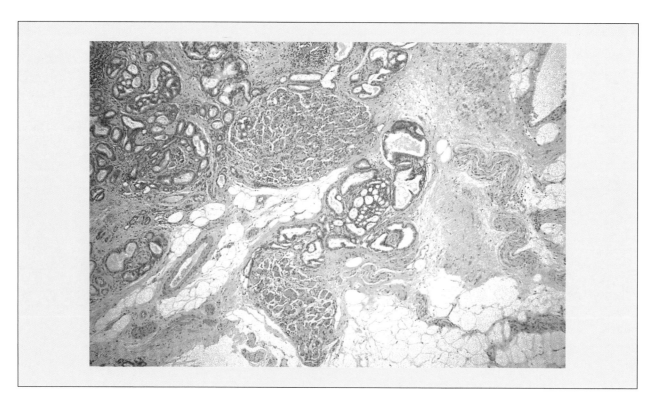

Figure 81   An adenocarcinoma can be seen extending posterolaterally beyond the gland into adipose tissue to encircle the neighboring nerves and ganglia. Perineural invasion must be considered during nerve-sparing surgery

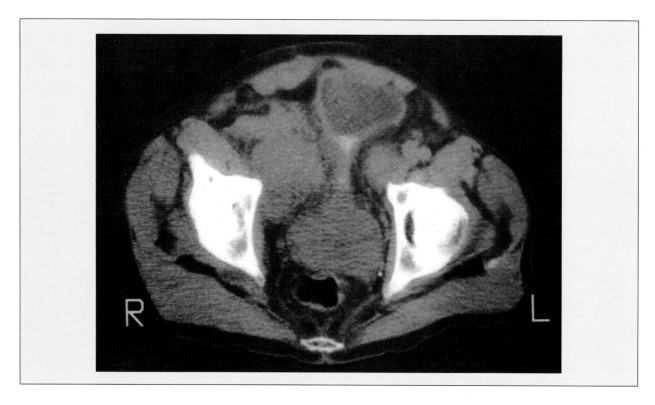

Figure 82   Locally advanced-stage T3/T4 prostate cancers may occasionally impinge posteriorly in the rectum to produce symptoms of tenesmus, constipation and, less commonly, rectal bleeding

15

Metastatic spread of prostate cancer

The most favored sites of prostate cancer metastases (Figure 83) are the obturator lymph nodes and the bony skeleton, especially the lumbosacral spine and pelvis. However, lymph nodes elsewhere, the lungs and other soft tissues may also be involved (Figures 84 and 85).

The reasons for the particular proclivity of prostate cancer metastases to develop in the skeleton have recently been elucidated[35,36]:

(1) Metastatic tumor cells release humoral factors, such as parathyroid hormone and interleukin-6,

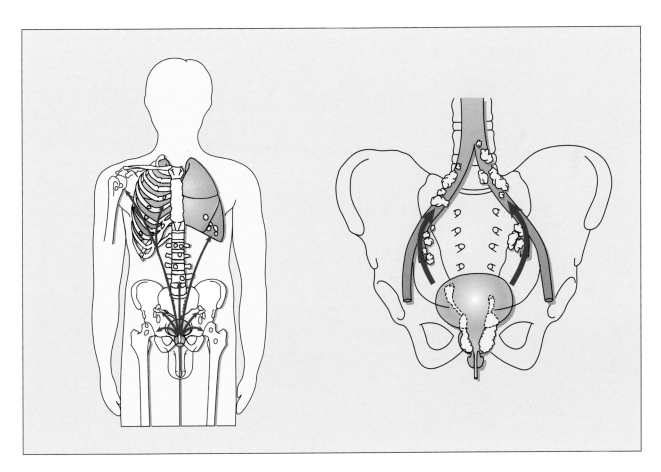

Figure 83   The favored sites of metastases from prostate cancer are the lymphatic nodes of the obturator fossa and the bony skeleton, in particular, the lumbosacral spine and bony pelvis

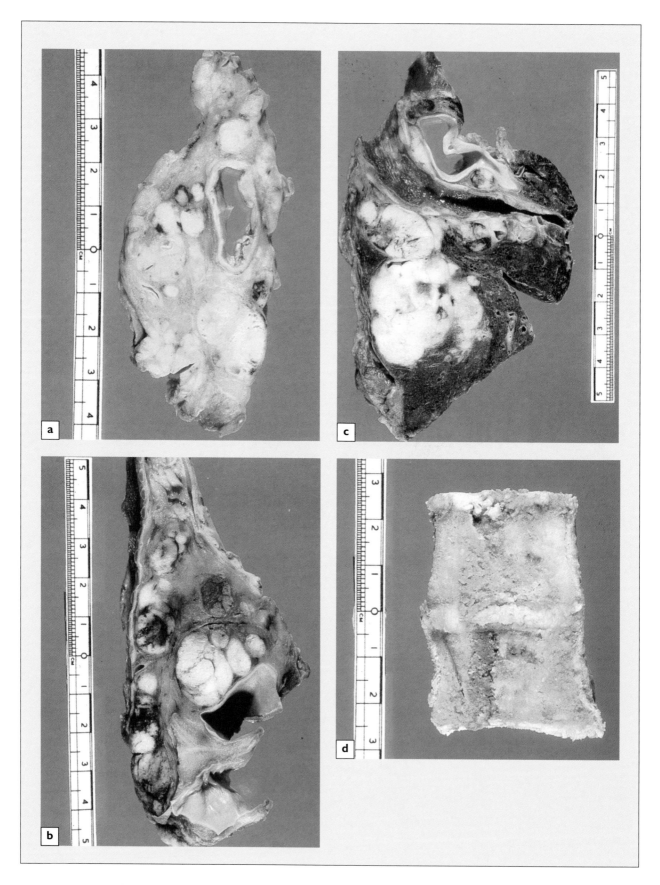

Figure 84   These specimens are the result of metastatic spread of prostate cancer to the lymph nodes in the pelvis and abdomen (a) and mediastinum (b), and to the lung (c) and spinal vertebrae (d)

that stimulate osteoclastic recruitment and differentiation.

(2) Prostate cancer cells concomitantly produce soluble paracrine factors such as transforming growth factor-β and insulin-like growth factor.

(3) Osteoclastic activity releases growth factors such as transforming growth factor-β that stim-ulate tumor growth, perpetuating the vicious cycle of excessive bone resorption.

(4) Osteoblastic activation in turn releases uniden-tified osteoblastic growth factors that also stim-ulate tumor cell growth, contributing to the cycle of abnormal bone formation (see Figure 35).

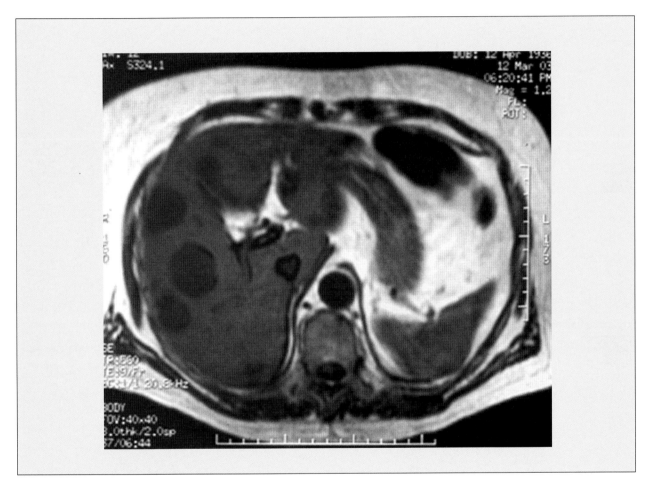

Figure 85   Multiple liver metastases due to metastatic adenocarcinoma of the prostate demonstrated by CT scan-ning in a patient with hormone-independent prostate cancer

16

Acute and chronic prostatitis

The inflammatory process in the prostate nearly always remains localized to the gland itself, although pyrexia and general malaise are not infrequently encountered. Acute prostatitis may progress to abscess formation, and the lesion may point and eventually drain either per urethra or per rectum. Chronic prostatitis mainly involves the peripheral zone of the prostate, but the inflammation may spread to involve the transitional zone and central zone as well (Figure 86).

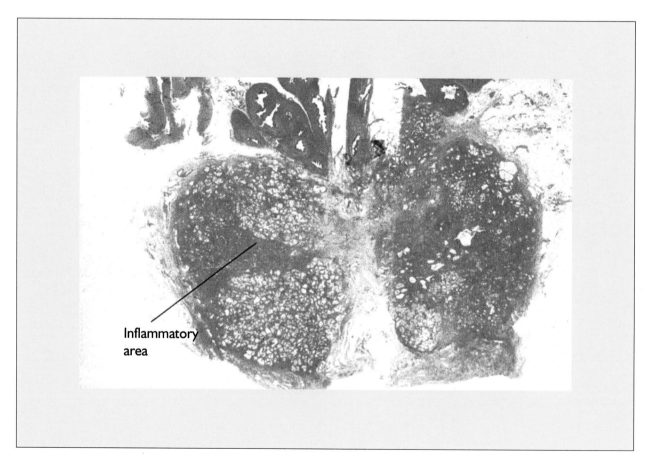

Inflammatory area

Figure 86   This abscess in the prostate is the result of untreated prostatitis. Such a focus of inflammation would also be easily discernible macroscopically (H & E)

17

Diagnosis of prostatic diseases

HISTORY

Because the prostate surrounds the urethra, patients who have prostatic diseases most frequently complain of micturition-related symptoms. These have been subdivided into irritative (storage) and obstructive (voiding) symptoms. Irritative symptoms have the most impact on the patient's quality of life.

To quantitate the severity of symptoms, a numerical symptom-scoring system was first devised by a subcommittee of the American Urological Association (AUA)[37,38] and then adopted by the International Consensus Committee (ICC) as the International Prostate Symptom Score (IPSS; Figure 87). As an adjunct to the symptom score, there is also

Urinary symptoms						
	not at all	less than 1 time in 5	less than half the time	about half the time	more than half the time	almost always
Over the past month or so, how often have you had a sensation of not emptying your bladder completely after you finished urinating?	[0]	[1]	[2]	[3]	[4]	[5]
Over the past month or so, how often have you had to urinate again less than two hours after you finished urinating?	[0]	[1]	[2]	[3]	[4]	[5]
Over the past month or so, how often have you found you stopped and started again several times when you urinated?	[0]	[1]	[2]	[3]	[4]	[5]
Over the past month or so, how often have you found it difficult to postpone urination?	[0]	[1]	[2]	[3]	[4]	[5]
Over the past month or so, how often have you had a weak urinary stream?	[0]	[1]	[2]	[3]	[4]	[5]
Over the past month or so, how often have you had to push or strain to begin urination?	[0]	[1]	[2]	[3]	[4]	[5]
Over the last month, how many times did you most typically get up to urinate from the time you went to bed at night until the time you got up in the morning?						
[0] none [1] 1 time [2] 2 times [3] 3 times [4] 4 times [5] 5 or more times						

Figure 87   The International Prostate Symptom Score (IPSS) is derived from the responses to these seven questions

a single question that attempts to evaluate the impact of the symptoms on the quality of life.

Other symptoms that are suggestive of either prostatic or bladder disease, but which are not encompassed by the IPSS, include perineal pain, hematuria, hemospermia and, in the case of metastatic prostate cancer, sudden onset of lower back or pelvic pain.

PHYSICAL EXAMINATION

A general physical examination, including blood pressure measurement, is important in patients with prostatic disease, as men beyond middle age not uncommonly harbor other co-morbid conditions such as hypertension, diabetes or chronic obstructive airways disease. A focused neurological examination will identify most significant neurological diseases, which may masquerade as lower urinary tract pathology. Palpation and percussion of the lower abdomen may reveal a chronically over-distended bladder due to chronic urinary retention.

The cornerstone of the physical examination in the patient with suspected prostatic disease is the digital rectal examination (DRE). This may be performed with the patient in the left lateral, knee–elbow or forward-bend position. A well-lubricated gloved finger is inserted into the rectum to evaluate the size and consistency of the gland.

The normal prostate should be the size of a chestnut and possess a springy consistency similar to that of the tip of the nose. The median sulcus is normally palpable, but the seminal vesicles should not be appreciable (Figure 88).

In prostatitis, the prostate may feel normal, boggy, tender or indurated on DRE. If a prostatic abscess is present, the gland becomes fluctuant and exquisitely tender. In benign prostatic hyperplasia, the prostate is usually symmetrically enlarged and maintains its normal springy consistency. Bimanual examination in a relaxed patient may sometimes reveal either an unsuspected intravesical component of benign prostatic hyperplasia or a chronically distended bladder.

DRE in patients with prostate cancer may reveal a distinct nodule, diffuse induration or asymmetry of the gland. When the lesion involves the seminal vesicles, these structures may become palpable as firm 'cords' running superolaterally from the indurated prostate itself[39].

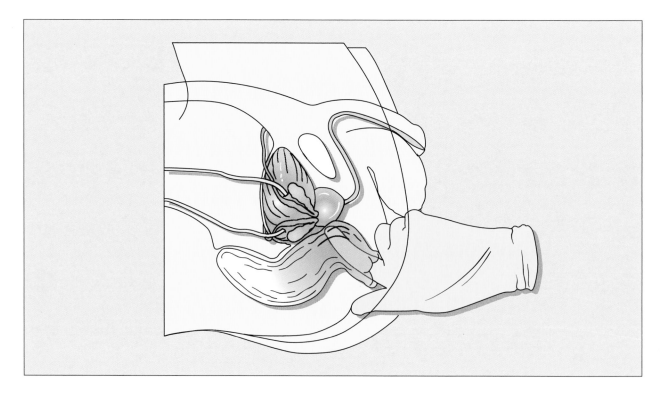

Figure 88   Digital rectal examination (DRE) allows the detection of posteriorly located tumors, which may be identified as an induration or distinct nodules, or as a cause of asymmetry of the gland

MICROSCOPY AND CULTURE OF URINE, AND EXPRESSED PROSTATIC SECRETIONS

Urine microscopy and culture are important in most patients with lower urinary tract symptoms. Hematuria on microscopy may alert the clinician to coincidental pathology such as transitional cell carcinoma or carcinoma-*in-situ*. In such cases, urine cytology and cystoscopy, as well as bladder biopsy, are indicated. A positive urine culture with antibiotic sensitivities indicates the need for appropriate antibiotic therapy.

If prostatitis is suspected, culture and microscopy of expressed prostatic secretions (EPS) are appropriate. The specimens must be carefully obtained (Figure 89) and bacteriological techniques capable of

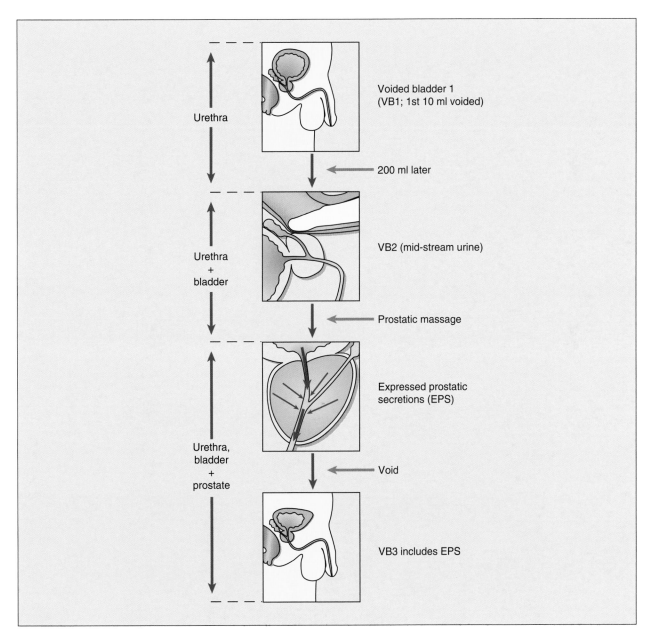

Figure 89 Bacterial prostatitis may be diagnosed by a lower tract localization (LTL) test. Initial and mid-stream urine specimens are collected and cultured; this is followed by a vigorous prostatic massage, after which an expressed prostatic secretion (EPS) sample is sent for culture. Finally, a further initial urine specimen is obtained and cultured. Differential bacterial counts among the various specimens may be an indication of an intraprostatic infection

quantifying small numbers of fastidious organisms, including facultative anaerobes such as *Ureaplasma urealyticum*, should be employed.

When the bladder urine is sterile, or nearly so, urethral colonization is indicated by a much higher count in the first-voided 10 ml of urine (voided bladder 1; VB1) than obtained from either EPS or the first-voided 10 ml of urine after prostatic massage (VB3). In contrast, with bacterial prostatitis, the bacterial count in the EPS and VB3 cultures should exceed those of the VB1 and mid-stream (VB2) cultures by at least a factor of 10 or more.

SEROLOGY

A blood urea nitrogen (BUN) and serum creatinine assay are sometimes requested in patients presenting with lower urinary tract symptoms. Around one in ten patients with benign prostatic hyperplasia and/or prostate cancer have some elevation of serum creatinine, although this is seldom the result of bladder outlet obstruction *per se*. A full blood count occasionally reveals anemia or other clinically significant abnormalities such as leukocytosis.

The most important – and most controversial – serological test in prostatic disease is the PSA assay. Levels of this glycoprotein (Figure 90) are elevated by any disease that interferes with the integrity of the basement membrane surrounding prostatic acini. In around one in ten patients with benign prostatic hyperplasia, in the occasional patient with prostatitis or prostatic infarction (Figure 91) and in most patients with clinically significant volumes of prostate cancer, PSA values are greater than the upper limit of normal (4 ng/ml[40,41] with the most commonly employed Hybritech™ or Abbott IMX™ immunometric assays).

Recently, it has been confirmed that differential assays comparing the ratio of free to complexed PSA may further help to discriminate between benign prostatic hyperplasia and prostate cancer[42] (Figure 92). As mentioned previously, in patients with prostate cancer, a greater proportion of the serum PSA is bound to the protein antichymotrypsin than in benign prostatic hyperplasia, resulting in a reduction of the free-to-total PSA ratio. The generally accepted cut-off point for the free-to-total PSA is 0.15.

Elevated total levels of PSA or reduction of the free-to-total PSA ratio below 0.15 may therefore act as a marker for as yet impalpable prostate cancer. In men whose life expectancy exceeds 10 years, earlier diagnosis of prostate cancer may allow curative treatment, and thus prevent local progression and/or the

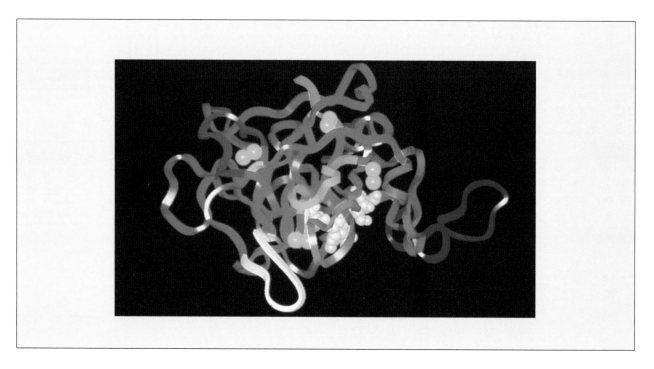

Figure 90   A three-dimensional model of the structure of the prostate-specific antigen (PSA) molecule

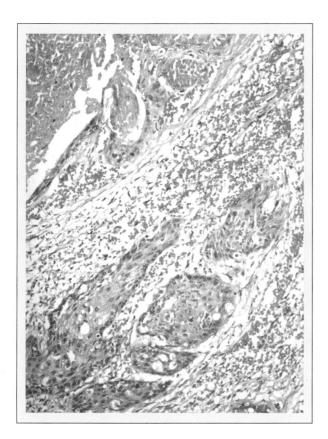

Figure 91   This histological section shows an area of prostatic infarction (upper left) with characteristic squamous metaplasia of the adjacent acini. Prostatic infarction is associated with a rise in PSA and, occasionally, with the development of acute urinary retention (H & E)

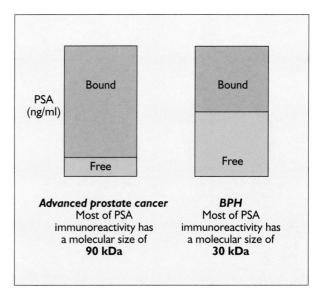

Figure 92   The ratio of free to total prostate-specific antigen (PSA) is greater in benign prostatic hyperplasia (BPH) than in prostate cancer. With the use of a highly sensitive immunofluoro-metric assay, the concentration of serum-free PSA in relation to PSA bound to the protein antichy-motrypsin can be determined, which may help to differentiate between these two prostatic diseases

development of metastases. Theoretically at least, this should reduce cancer-specific mortality, although this remains to be proved by long-term randomized studies of screening and early intervention. Currently, the jury is still out in respect to organized PSA screening of asymptomatic men, but many informed individuals make the choice for themselves and request annual PSA testing as part of a more general screening examination.

IMAGING STUDIES AND URINARY FLOW RATE DETERMINATION

The combined use of imaging studies and uroflow measurement aims to identify both structural and functional abnormalities in the upper and lower urinary tract. The normal bladder fills from undilated kidneys and ureters to a volume of around 300–500 ml and then empties completely through an unobstructed outlet, at a maximum flow rate of more than 15 ml/s. A plain X-ray will identify radio-opaque calculi in the bladder (Figure 93).

Contrast administered intravenously may demonstrate anatomical abnormalities in the upper tracts and, albeit with less sensitivity, in the bladder itself. Figure 94 is an intravenous urogram (IVU) showing the typical IVU appearances of a large, benignly enlarged, prostate causing an indentation at the base of the bladder. In a small minority of cases, the outflow obstruction due to benign prostatic hyperplasia is severe enough to result in bilateral hydronephrosis (Figure 95). In contrast, in locally advanced prostate cancer, unilateral or bilateral ureteric obstruction is not uncommon and may be the result of either obstruction of the intramural ureter at the level of the trigone or constriction at the pelvic brim due to lymph node metastases (Figure 96).

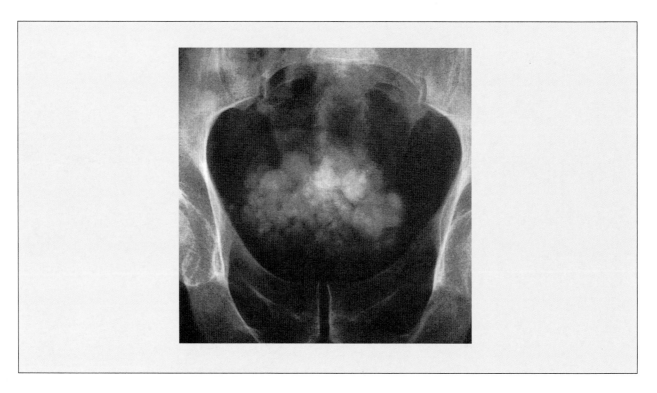

Figure 93   These multiple bladder stones, visualized on a plain abdominal X-ray, are seen in association with a benignly enlarged prostate

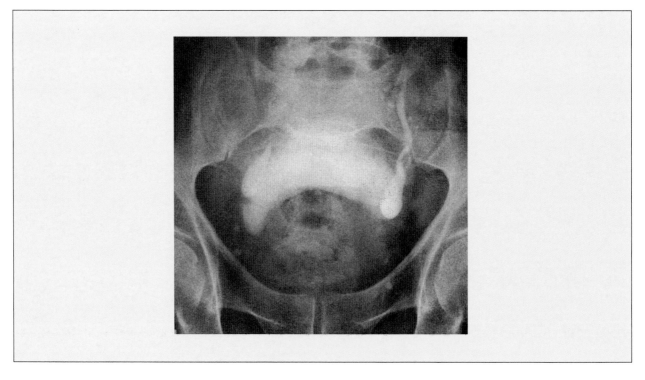

Figure 94   This intravenous urogram shows a benign prostate gland which is sufficiently massive as to cause an indentation of the base of the bladder. The adenoma weighed more than 200 g at the time of removal by retropubic prostatectomy

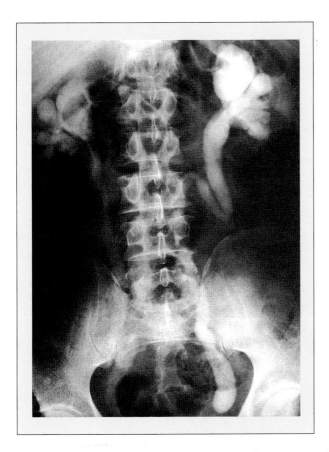

Figure 95 An intravenous urogram showing bilateral hydronephrosis secondary to benign prostatic hyperplasia. The distal ends of the ureters are characteristically hook-shaped in appearance

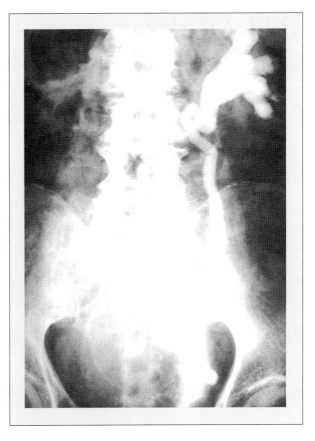

Figure 96 Nephrostogram showing lower ureteric obstruction and hydronephrosis secondary to prostatic adenocarcinoma

TRANSABDOMINAL ULTRASOUND IMAGING

Transabdominal ultrasound imaging provides a simple, non-invasive and cost-effective means of imaging the bladder and prostate, and excludes upper tract dilatation. Pre- and post-void estimations of bladder volume allow evaluation of the post-void residual (PVR) volume of urine, although several studies have shown that there is a marked void-to-void variation in the values recorded[43]. Median lobe enlargement of the prostate is readily visualized (Figure 97), but the architecture of the posterior portion and transitional zone of the gland is best imaged by an endocavity transrectal ultrasound probe. Bladder calculi are also visible using this technology.

UROFLOWMETRY

Uroflowmetry is capable of quantitating objectively the severity of the bladder outflow obstruction. A voided volume of more than 150 ml is required to achieve a reliable recording. With this proviso, the test has an acceptable test–retest reproducibility[44]. Patients should be advised to avoid abdominal straining during the measurement, as this may result in artefactual peaks, and should feel that the bladder is full prior to the test. Figures 98 and 99 are examples of a normal uroflow trace and an obstructed uroflow trace, respectively.

Maximum uroflow values are the most clinically useful single parameter. Values above 15 ml/s have an approximately 70% probability of obstruction, whereas values below 10 ml/s are associated with a

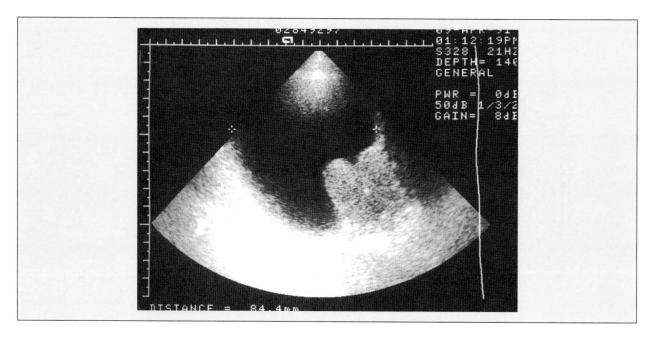

Figure 97   Transabdominal ultrasound showing pronounced indentation of the bladder due to considerable benign prostatic hyperplasia

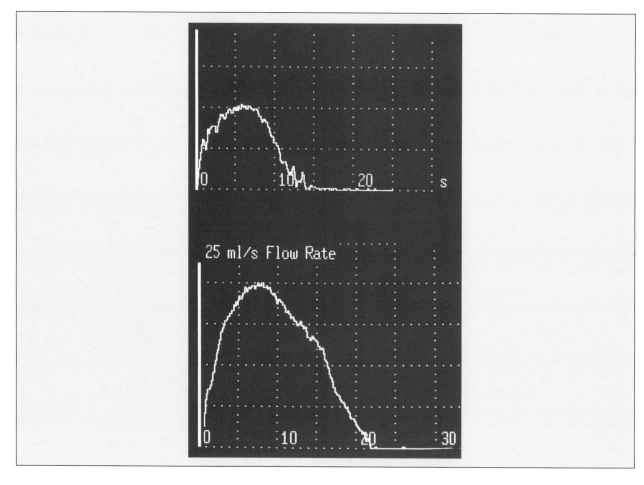

Figure 98   These two uroflowmetry recordings were both taken in the same unobstructed patient, one at a volume of 100 ml, the other with a voided volume of 350 ml. The apparent discrepancy demonstrates the dependence of uroflow measurements on adequate prevoiding bladder filling

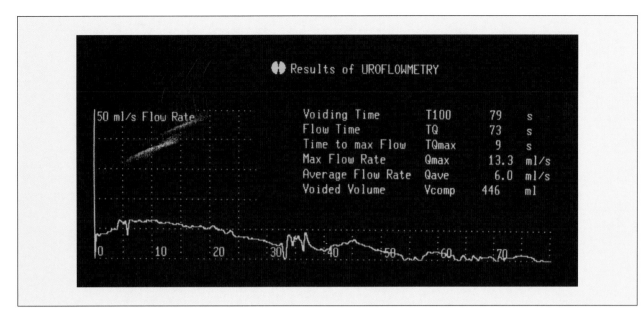

Figure 99   This uroflow recording from a patient with bladder outflow obstruction secondary to benign prostatic hyperplasia shows a reduced maximum flow and prolonged voiding

urodynamic bladder outlet obstruction in more than 90% of cases. Typically, men with lower urinary tract symptoms that are the result of an overactive bladder rather than bladder outlet obstruction due to benign prostatic enlargement have normal or supranormal flow patterns.

PRESSURE-FLOW URODYNAMICS

Pressure-flow urodynamics is the term used for the investigation that involves measurement of intravesical pressure during filling and voiding and urinary flow rate. This is achieved by the insertion of a filling catheter and pressure recording device into the bladder, usually by the transurethral route, but sometimes by suprapubic puncture. To discount the effect of abdominal straining and thereby assess the impact of genuine bladder contractions, another small tube is inserted into the rectum and this pressure is subtracted from the intravesical pressure. The normal bladder should accommodate up to 300–500 ml of fluid without undue pressure rise. As a response to prostatic obstruction, bladder compliance is reduced and involuntary contractions occur during filling. During voiding, bladder pressures are typically high and flow rates low. When late-stage bladder outflow obstruction occurs, and in conditions such as diabetic neuropathy, bladder contractions are impaired and a low-pressure, low-flow

scenario develops. Urodynamics provide the only reliable way of confirming this diagnosis.

TRANSRECTAL ULTRASOUND IMAGING

Transrectal ultrasound (TRUS) imaging of the prostate serves several purposes:

- Imaging the internal architecture of the gland and periprostatic tissues, including seminal vesicles;

- Estimation of prostate volume;

- Facilitation and targeting of ultrasound-guided prostate biopsy.

A 7-MHz endocavity ultrasound probe is commonly used and the prostate viewed in both anteroposterior and sagittal planes (Figures 100 and 101). Benign prostatic hyperplasia is characterized by hypoechoic expansion of the transitional zone[45] (Figure 102). Adenocarcinomata may sometimes be visualized as hypoechoic foci (and less often as hyperechoic), most usually located in the peripheral zone (Figures 103 and 104) and less frequently at the apex of the gland[46] (Figure 105). Many smaller prostate cancers, however, are isoechoic and can be identified only by systematic sextant biopsy.

On occasion, TRUS allows estimation of the local stage of a prostate cancer because asymmetry and

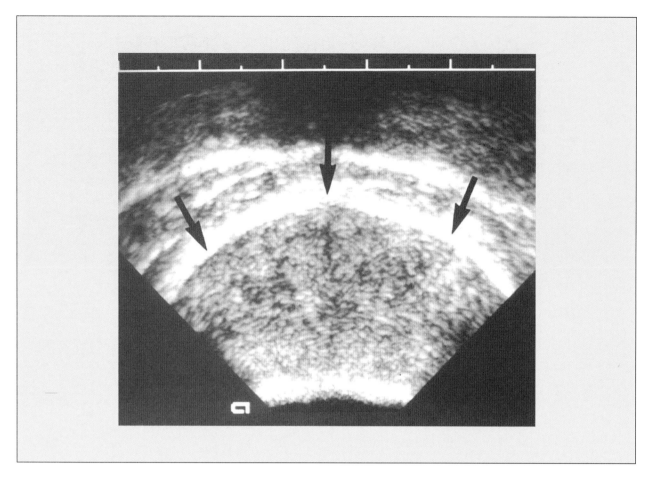

Figure 100   Transrectal ultrasound showing the appearances of the normal prostate in the anteroposterior view

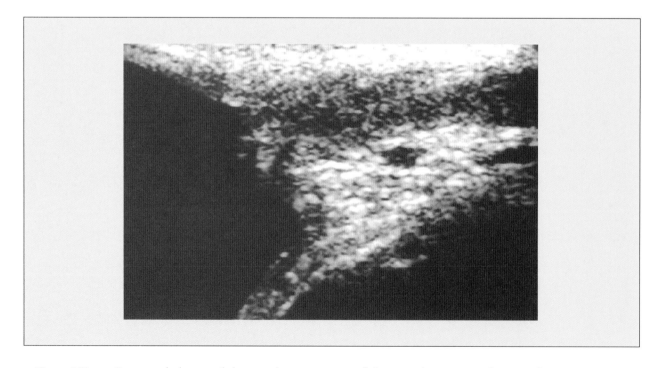

Figure 101   Transrectal ultrasound showing the appearances of the normal prostate in the sagittal view

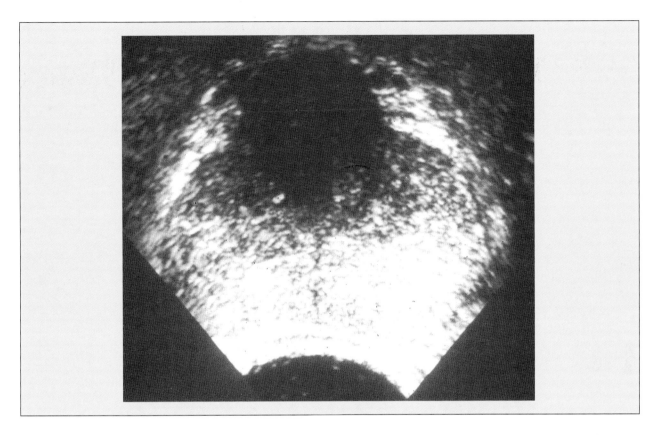

Figure 102   Transrectal ultrasound of a prostate with considerable benign prostatic hyperplasia showing a characteristically large periurethral hypoechoic area (anteroposterior view)

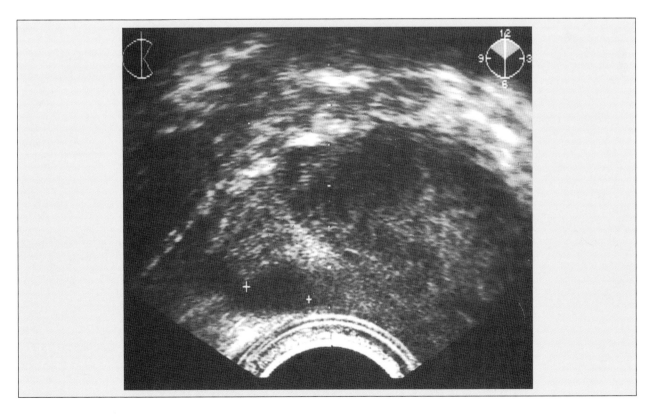

Figure 103   Transrectal ultrasound showing a hypoechoic area in the peripheral zone which proved, on biopsy, to be an adenocarcinoma (anteroposterior view)

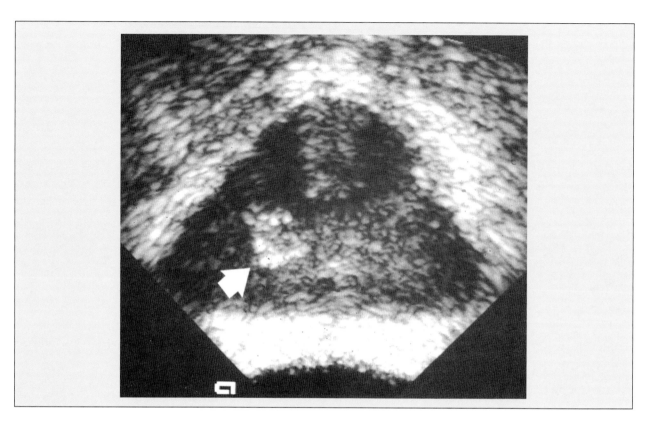

Figure 104   Transrectal ultrasound showing an atypical hyperechoic appearance (arrowed) of prostate cancer

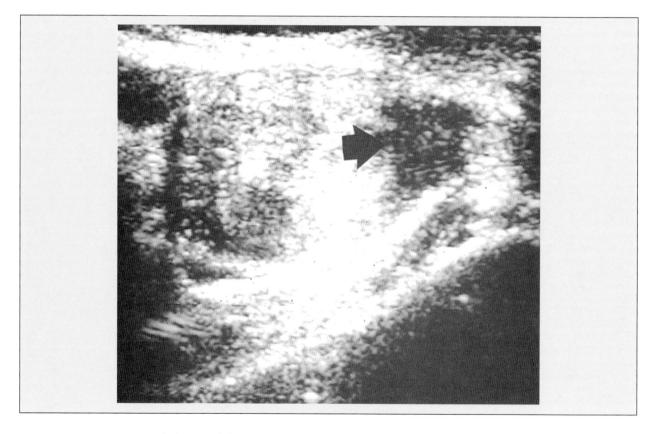

Figure 105   Transrectal ultrasound showing a hypoechoic adenocarcinoma at the apex of the gland (arrowed)

irregularity of the capsule are associated with extra-capsular spread of adenocarcinoma[47].

The advent of color Doppler ultrasound imaging and its incorporation into TRUS technology have allowed the evaluation of prostatic blood flow. The main clinical value of this technology is in the imaging of patients with prostatitis, when objective confirmation of the inflammatory process may be helpful (Figure 106). Prostatic calculi, which may be the cause of prostatic inflammation, can often be visualized (Figure 107), sometimes as a cause of obstruction to the ejaculatory ducts.

After administration of a covering dose of an antibiotic treatment, which should be continued for several days, systematic TRUS-guided biopsy of the prostate may be obtained (Figure 108) under local anesthesia[48]. Sextant or octant (sometimes as many as 12) biopsies are taken, together with guided biopsy of any suspicious foci, using an automated biopsy needle[49]. The tissue specimens are subsequently carefully analyzed histologically[50] (Figure 109).

COMPUTED TOMOGRAPHY AND MAGNETIC RESONANCE IMAGING

Computed tomography (CT) and magnetic resonance imaging (MRI) are sometimes helpful in the staging of prostatic cancer. Less frequently, these technologies are used to establish the precise volume of benign prostatic hyperplasia present[51].

CT scanning reveals the dimensions of the prostate, but does not clearly demonstrate its internal architecture (Figure 110). Irregularity of the gland may suggest the presence of extracapsular extension of tumor, but the sensitivity and specificity of this observation are low. CT scans are also employed to identify pelvic lymphadenopathy, usually an indication of metastatic spread but, even in such a situation, the accuracy is still low. In equivocal cases, CT guidance may allow fine-needle aspiration of enlarged lymph nodes for confirmatory cytological study (Figure 111).

Whole-body coils allow MRI imaging of the prostate, with which the peripheral zone may be

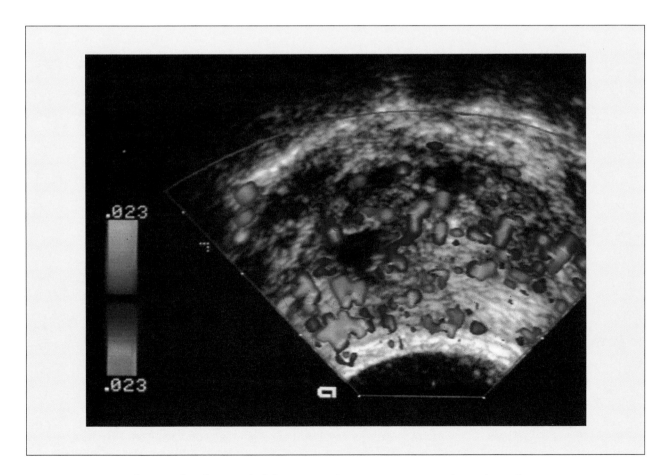

Figure 106 Color Doppler ultrasound of the prostate demonstrating increased vascularity due to acute prostatitis

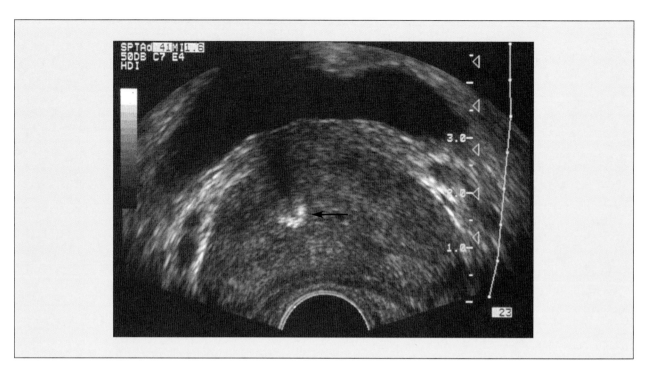

Figure 107   Transrectal ultrasound showing a prostatic calculus (arrowed) as a white patch. The calculus blocks the transmission of ultrasound waves, resulting in characteristic acoustic shadowing

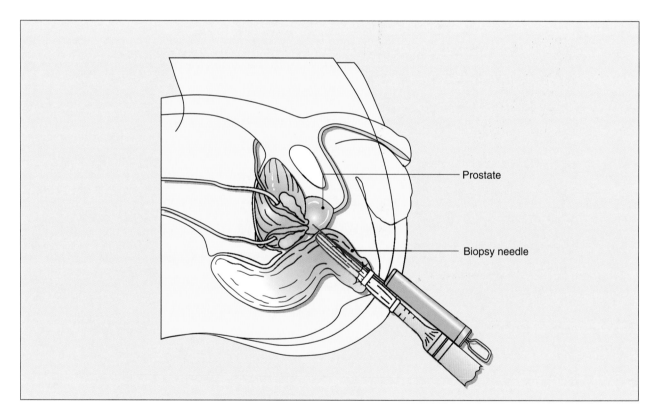

Figure 108   The procedure for transrectal ultrasound-guided biopsy of the prostate should always be carried out under antibiotic cover, which should be continued for 3–4 days post-biopsy to reduce the incidence of infective complications. At present, the most common indications for biopsy are either an elevated prostate-specific antigen (PSA) or a prostate that feels abnormal on digital rectal examination

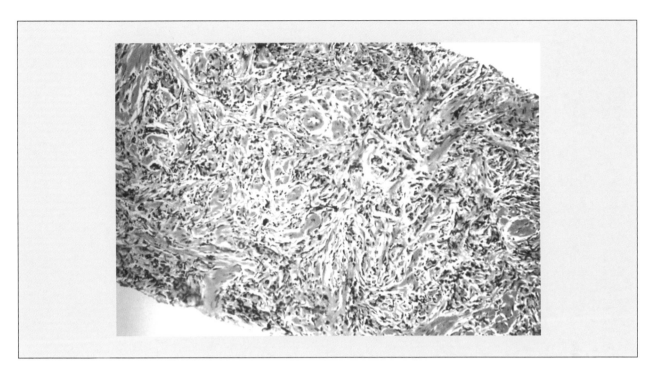

Figure 109   A prostate biopsy specimen, taken with the use of an automated transrectal ultrasound-guided biopsy device, reveals poorly differentiated adenocarcinoma (H & E)

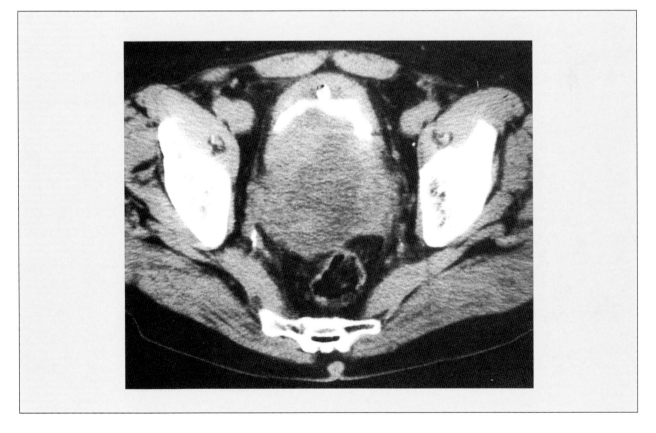

Figure 110   Although computed tomography scanning is able to demonstrate the prostate, visualization of the internal architecture is poor. Also, the use of this imaging modality for local staging is limited

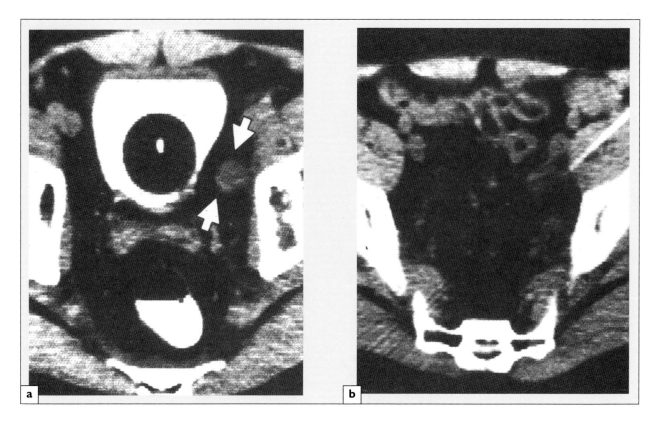

Figure 111   Computed tomography scanning can reveal pelvic lymphadenopathy (a), albeit with limited specificity, and can also be used to guide fine-needle aspiration (b) for cytological examination

distinguished from the transitional zone (Figure 112). Adenocarcinoma may also be visualized by this means, although not all prostate cancers are as clearly demarcated from normal tissue as the example shown in Figure 113.

Endorectal MRI provides more architectural detail of internal prostatic anatomy[52]. Figures 114 and 115 show T_1- and T_2-weighted images, respectively, of a prostate expanded by benign prostatic hyperplasia tissue. Figure 116 is an MRI scan, taken with an endorectal coil, of a lesion in the peripheral zone of the prostate that lies close to, and probably involves, the neurovascular bundle on the affected side.

MRI may also be useful in demonstrating lymph node metastases (Figure 117), or involvement of the spine (Figure 118), pelvis or long bones.

As MRI technology is advancing rapidly, we may anticipate even more precise and discriminatory images in the future. The use of enhancing agents such as gadolinium has already improved results, but these advances have yet to be translated into clinically useful techniques.

RADIONUCLIDE BONE SCANNING

Technetium radionuclide bone scanning has transformed our ability to detect early bone metastases from prostate cancer[53]. This technology, which is able to demonstrate clearly the abnormal vascularity in skeletal metastases, has far higher sensitivity and specificity than the radiological skeletal surveys that it has now replaced.

Although bone scans are seldom positive in patients with PSA values below 20 ng/ml[54], they may be useful as a baseline in newly diagnosed cases because they allow documentation of false-positive areas due to other disease processes, such as osteoarthrosis of the spine or Paget's disease.

The most common appearance of prostate cancer metastases on a bone scan is as multiple 'hot spots', mainly affecting the lumbosacral spine and pelvis (Figures 119 and 120). The long bones and skull, however, may also be involved.

In very extensive metastatic disease, the bone scan may occasionally be misleading because of diffusely increased skeletal uptake of radionuclide, an appearance known as a 'superscan' (Figure 121).

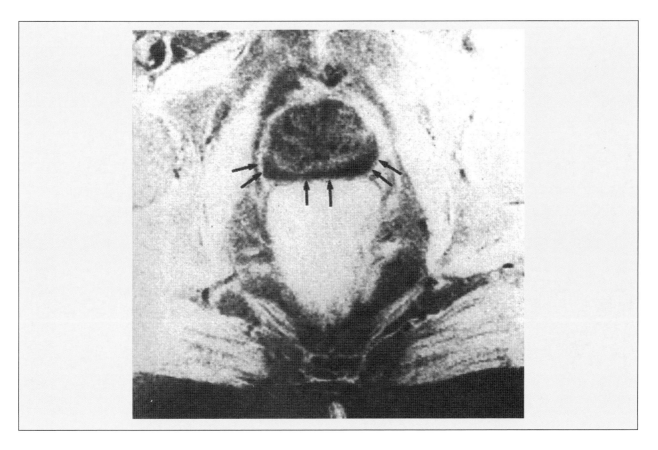

Figure 112   Magnetic resonance imaging scan, using an external body coil, allows differentiation of the peripheral zone (arrowed) from the hyperplastic transitional zone

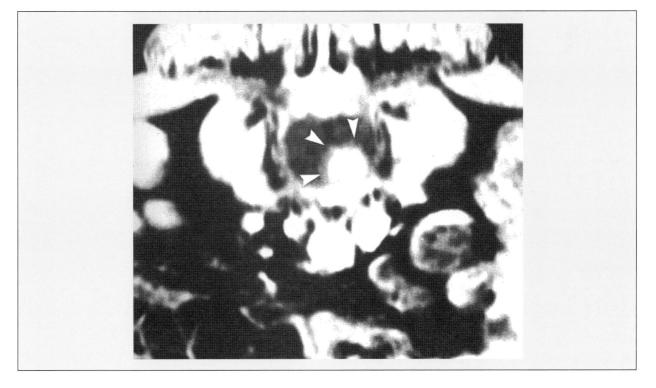

Figure 113   Magnetic resonance imaging scan, using an external body coil, shows a peripherally located prostatic adenocarcinoma (arrowed)

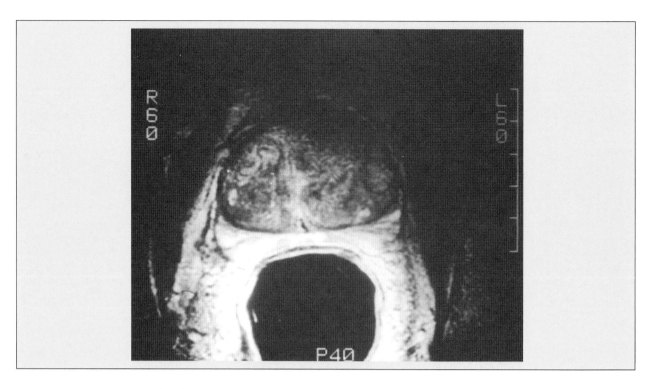

Figure 114   A T_1-weighted magnetic resonance imaging scan, using an endorectal imaging coil, reveals an enlarged prostate showing changes of benign prostatic hyperplasia

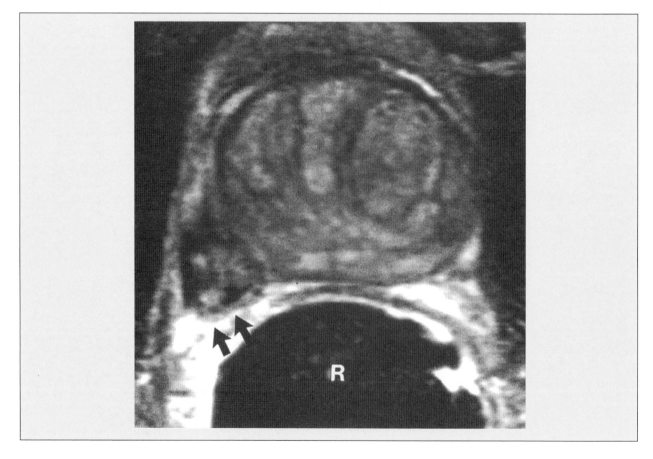

Figure 115   A T_2-weighted magnetic resonance imaging scan, using an endorectal coil, reveals a peripherally located prostatic adenocarcinoma (arrowed)

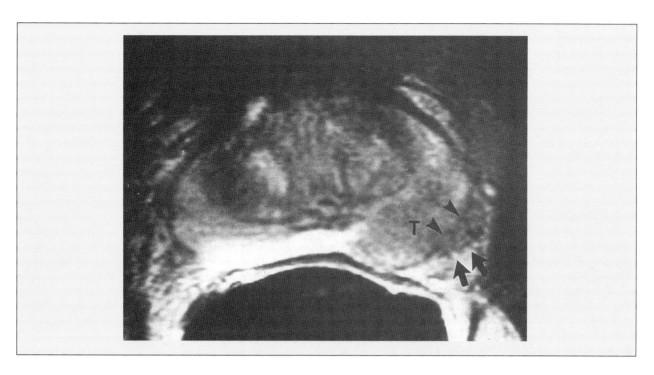

Figure 116   An endorectal magnetic resonance imaging scan showing a peripherally located adenocarcinoma (arrowed) involving the neurovascular bundle on that side

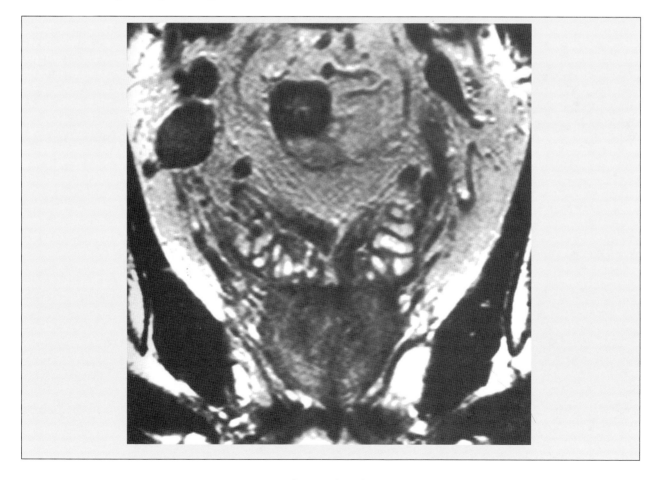

Figure 117   Magnetic resonance imaging scan showing lymph node enlargement (on the right) due to metastatic prostate cancer. The seminal vesicles are also visualized on this scan

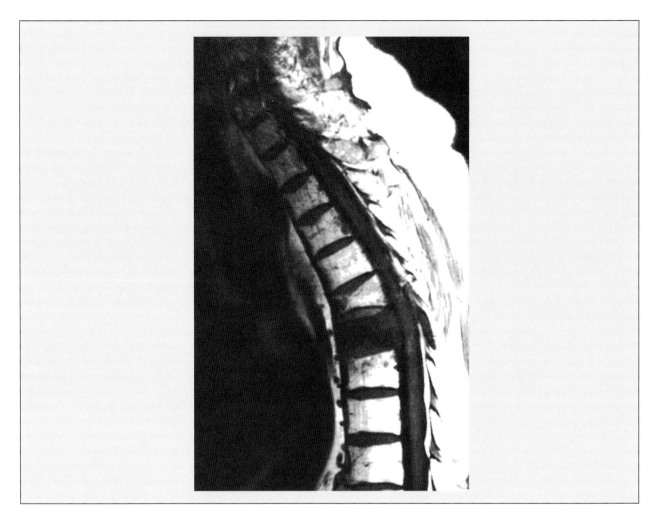

Figure 118   Magnetic resonance imaging scan of the thoracic spine showing involvement of one of the dorsal vertebral bodies by metastatic prostatic cancer. The adjacent vertebral body shows signs of collapse

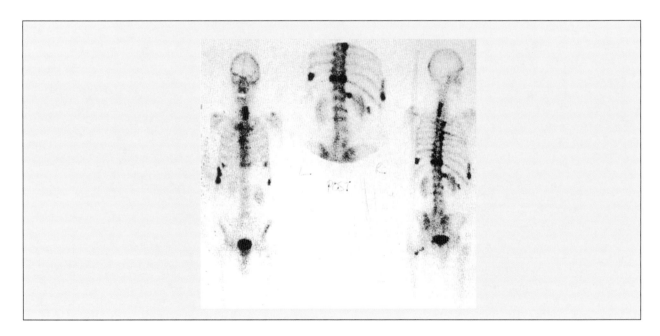

Figure 119   A radionuclide bone scan showing multiple metastatic deposits due to adenocarcinoma of the prostate

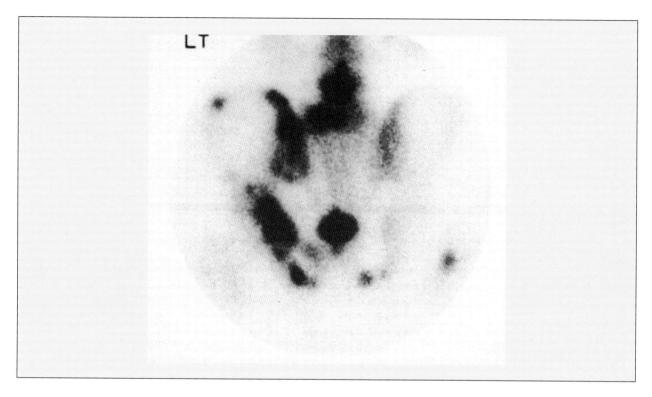

Figure 120   A radionuclide bone scan showing 'hot spots' in the pelvis and lumbar spine, an indication of metastatic prostate cancer

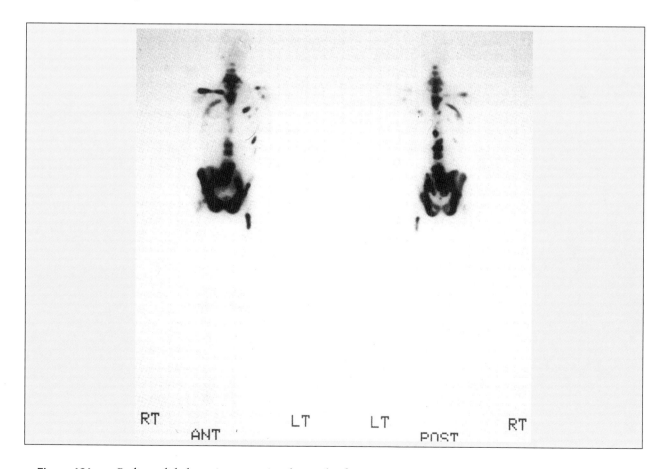

Figure 121   Radionuclide bone 'superscan' is the result of very extensive metastatic prostate cancer

18

Treatment options

BENIGN PROSTATIC HYPERPLASIA

Benign prostatic hyperplasia therapy has evolved over the last two decades from a simple choice between watchful waiting and transurethral resection of the prostate to more complex treatment decisions between various medical therapies and an expanding range of minimally invasive treatment options. Most patients who suffer some degree of bother from their benign prostatic hyperplasia-associated symptoms will now opt for medical therapy in the first instance. Plant extracts from a variety of sources (Figure 122) are popular, especially in continental Europe, but there is little hard evidence from randomized trials of their efficacy and safety. α-Blockers, such as doxazosin, tamsulosin and alfuzosin, can all be administered once per day and produce rapid and sustainable improvement of lower urinary tract symptoms and uroflow (Figure 123)[55]. It has been argued that tamsulosin, which has selec-

tivity for the α_{1A} and α_{1D} adrenoceptor subtypes, and alfuzosin, which is also relatively 'uroselective' (i.e. has more impact on prostate obstruction than blood pressure) have some advantages over doxazosin and terazosin, which have a balanced effect on all three receptor subtypes. However, doxazosin reduces the blood pressure in hypertensive men but has little or no impact on the blood pressure of normotensive individuals[56]. Doxazosin also reduces platelet adhesiveness and reduces LDL cholesterol, and thus may offer some cardiovascular protection in addition to improvement of lower urinary tract symptoms and uroflow[57]. Both doxazosin and terazosin, but not tamsulosin or alfuzosin, have been shown to cause apoptosis within the prostate, and it has been argued that this may rebalance the proliferative processes that underlie the condition (Figure 124). However, the clinical utility of this is still unproven.

American Dwarf Palm/Saw Palmetto	(fruits)	(Serenoa Repens/Sabal Serrulata)
African Plum tree	(barks)	(Pygom Africanum)
South African Star Grass, Pine, Spruce	(roots)	(Hypaxis Rooperi) (Pinus) (Picea)
Stinging nettle	(roots)	(Urtion Dioico)
Rye	(pollen)	(Secale Cereale)
Pumpkin	(seeds)	(Cucurbita Pepo)

Figure 122   Plant extracts are popular among patients for treatment of benign prostatic hyperplasia, especially in continental Europe. The names and origins of some of the more frequently used compounds are illustrated

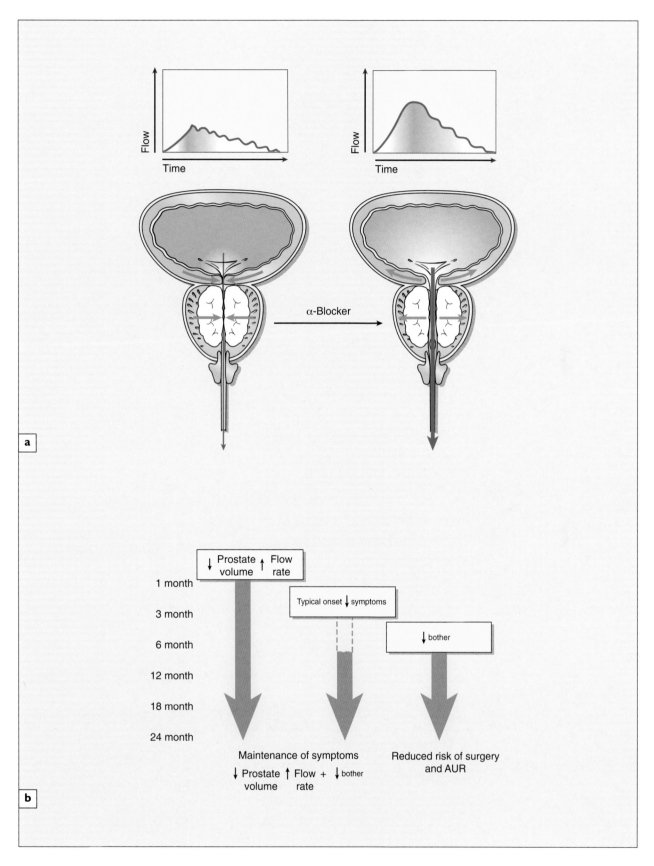

Figure 123   (a) α-Blocking agents relax the prostate and bladder neck and improve urinary flow rates and enhance bladder emptying. (b) Effects of 5α-reductase inhibitors. They offer lasting symptom relief and flow rate improvement and reduce the incidence of acute urinary retention (AUR) and surgery

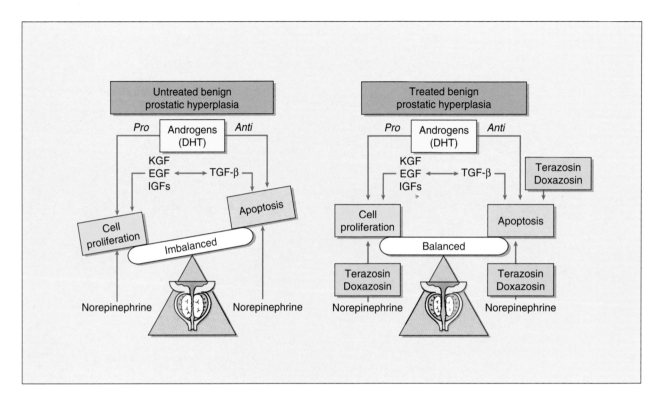

Figure 124   Benign prostatic hyperplasia results from an imbalance between stromal and epithelial proliferation and apoptosis. The α-blockers doxazosin and terazosin may exert some of their effect by restoring the balance between these opposing influences

The 5α-reductase type 2 inhibitor, finasteride, at a dose of 5 mg/day, effectively reduces prostate volume by around 20% and improves symptoms and uroflow almost to the same extent as the α-blockers, but only after a 3–6-month treatment period[58]. Available evidence suggests that finasteride works most effectively in men with a clinically enlarged prostate and a PSA value over 1.5 ng/ml; this effect is well maintained over 6 years of follow up. The Proscar Long-term Efficacy and Safety Study (PLESS) has demonstrated that finasteride can reduce benign prostatic hyperplasia-associated complications such as acute urinary retention and the need for prostate surgery by more than 50%[59]. This beneficial impact of medical therapy on benign prostatic hyperplasia progression has been confirmed by the Medical Therapy of Prostate Symptoms (MTOPS) study[60], which has been recently reported. In this 4.5-year trial, the combination of finasteride and doxazosin was significantly more effective than either agent alone or identical placebo in terms of preventing benign prostatic hyperplasia progression, defined as a 4-point or greater rise in symptom score, or development of acute retention or the need for benign prostatic hyperplasia-related surgery (Figures

125–127). The overall risk of progression, mostly due to symptomatic progression, was reduced by 39% for doxazosin, 34% for finasteride and 67% for combination therapy, respectively. The risk of acute retention was reduced by 31% for doxazosin, 67% for finasteride and 79% for combination therapy, while the risk of prostate-related surgery was reduced by 64% and 67%, respectively for finasteride and combination therapy, with no significant change in risk noted for the doxazosin group compared with placebo. The novel agent dutasteride can be distinguished from finasteride by its ability to inhibit both type 1 and type 2 isoforms of 5α-reductase. Recent data confirm that this compound also significantly improves lower urinary tract symptoms and uroflow in men with an enlarged prostate[61] with a side-effect profile rather similar to finasteride. Roehrborn and colleagues have confirmed that serum PSA can act as a surrogate for prostate volume[62], and that 5α-reductase inhibitors are used most effectively in men with PSA values > 1.5 ng/ml[63,64].

The different impacts of these various medical therapies for benign prostatic hyperplasia on sexual function should not be overlooked. A recent survey has found a strong association between the severity

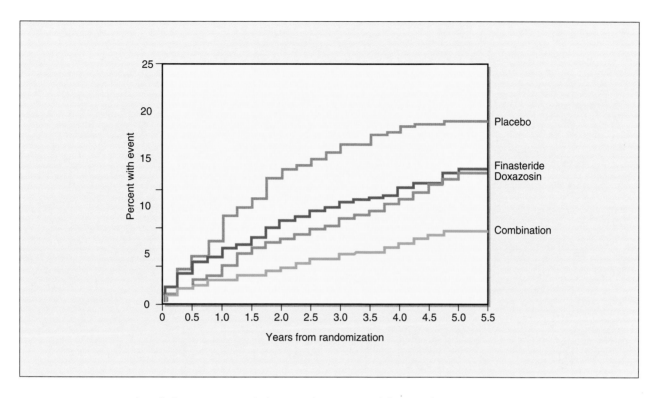

Figure 125   Results of the MTOPS trial showing the impact of finasteride, doxazosin, placebo, or combination therapy on progression of benign prostatic hyperplasia

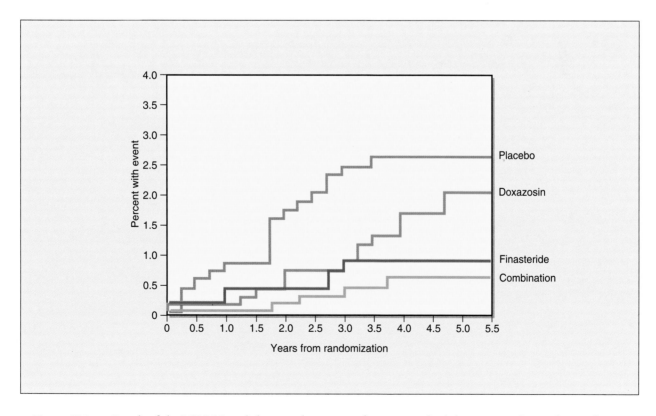

Figure 126   Result of the MTOPS trial showing the impact of various medical therapies on the incidence of acute urinary retention

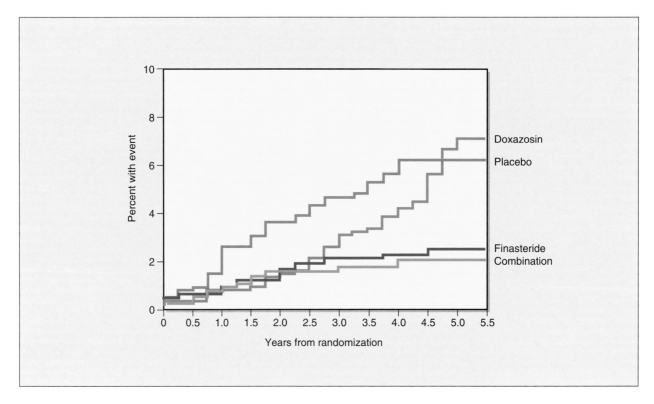

Figure 127   Results of the MTOPS trial showing the impact of various medical therapies on the need for benign prostatic hyperplasia-related invasive therapy

of lower urinary tract symptoms and sexual dysfunction[65]. While 5α-reductase inhibitors are associated with a loss of libido or the development of erectile dysfunction in 3–5% of patients[66], α-blockers have a more favorable impact on sexual function. Alfuzosin, in particular, has been reported to have a positive effect on sexual quality of life[67]. Tamsulosin, by contrast, seems to have little impact in this respect and has been reported to induce reversible retrograde ejaculation in up to 17% of subjects[68].

Surgical treatment options are now mainly employed in men who have failed to respond to medical therapy or in those suffering complications of benign prostatic hyperplasia such as acute urinary retention. Transurethral incision of the prostate (Figure 128) is only applicable to those with smaller prostates. Transurethral resection of the prostate, under either an epidural or a light general anesthesia, still constitutes the gold standard[69] (Figure 129). For men with gland volumes greater than 100 ml with severe symptoms and bother, an open prostatectomy, either by the retropubic (Figure 130) or the transvesical (Figure 131) route is still a useful option. However, newer technologies such as Holmium laser

resection with tissue morcellation[70] (Figure 132), interstitial laser therapy and microwave thermotherapy are all producing promising results, with possibly lower morbidity, especially in terms of bleeding. Most surgical approaches have a negative impact on ejaculation, but leave erections and sensation of orgasm unaffected[71]. This effect is not usually too troublesome provided that the patient has been counseled in advance. A minority of patients who undergo surgery for benign prostatic hyperplasia eventually develop recurrent lower urinary tract symptoms or hematuria. In these individuals, further investigations, including pressure-flow urodynamics and cystoscopy, are often necessary. The re-operation rate for transurethral resection of the prostate has been estimated at 2% per annum; however, it may be higher for some of the newer technologies. Finasteride has also been shown to be useful in the management of hematuria after transurethral resection of the prostate[72].

A decision diagram for the management of lower urinary tract symptom-associated benign prostatic hyperplasia in primary care is shown in Figure 133.

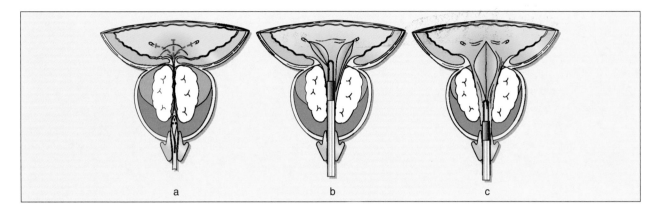

Figure 128   Transurethral incision of the prostate (TUIP). This technique is applicable to men with smaller prostates. Either a bilateral (a and b) or single incision (c) is made from the ureteric orifice to the verumontanum

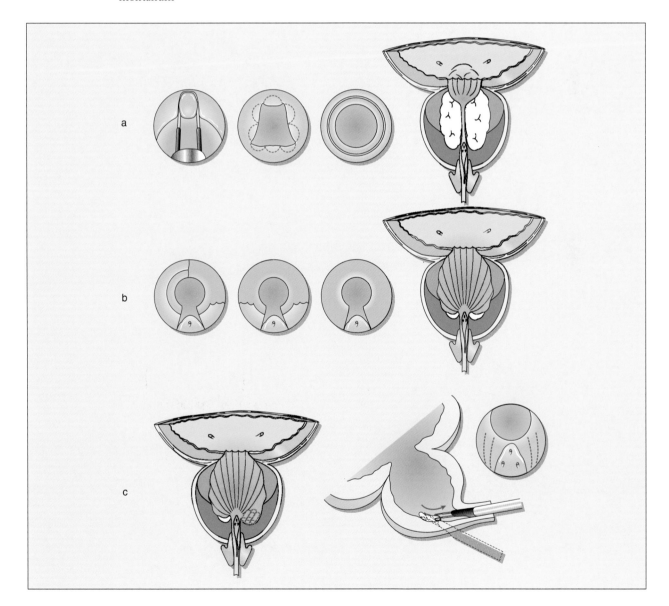

Figure 129   Transurethral resection of the prostate (TURP). The bladder neck, two lateral lobes and posterior portion of the prostate are resected as depicted, with careful preservation of the verumontanum

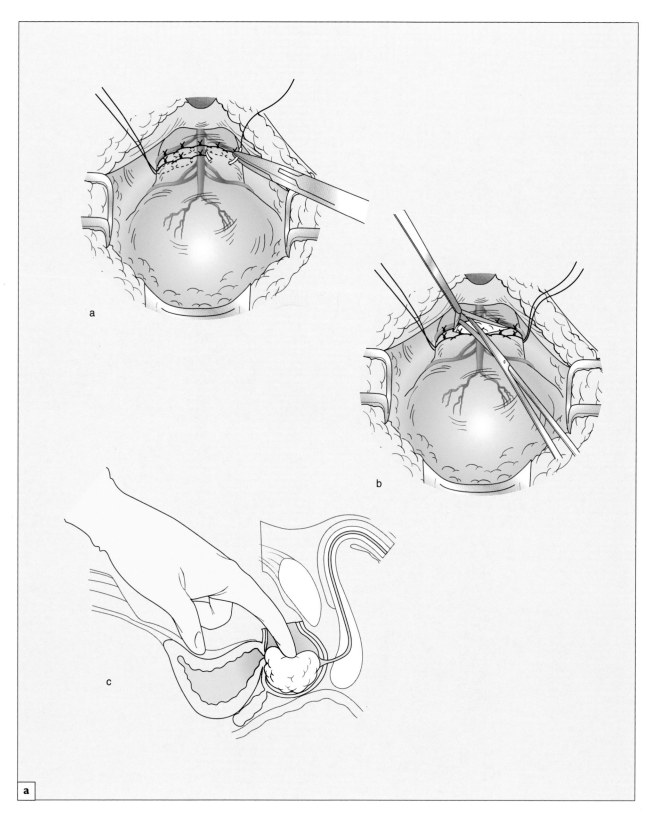

Figure 130   Retropubic prostatectomy: the prostate is exposed through a transverse lower abdominal incision. The anterior capsule is sutured to reduce blood loss (a) and then incised transversely (b). The transitional zone adenoma is enucleated digitally (c) and any adhesions divided with scissors, taking care not to damage the urethral sphincter (d). Two lateral sutures are placed and the bladder neck drawn down into the prostatic cavity with interrupted sutures (e). A urethral catheter is inserted and the anterior capsule closed with a running stitch (f) (*continued*)

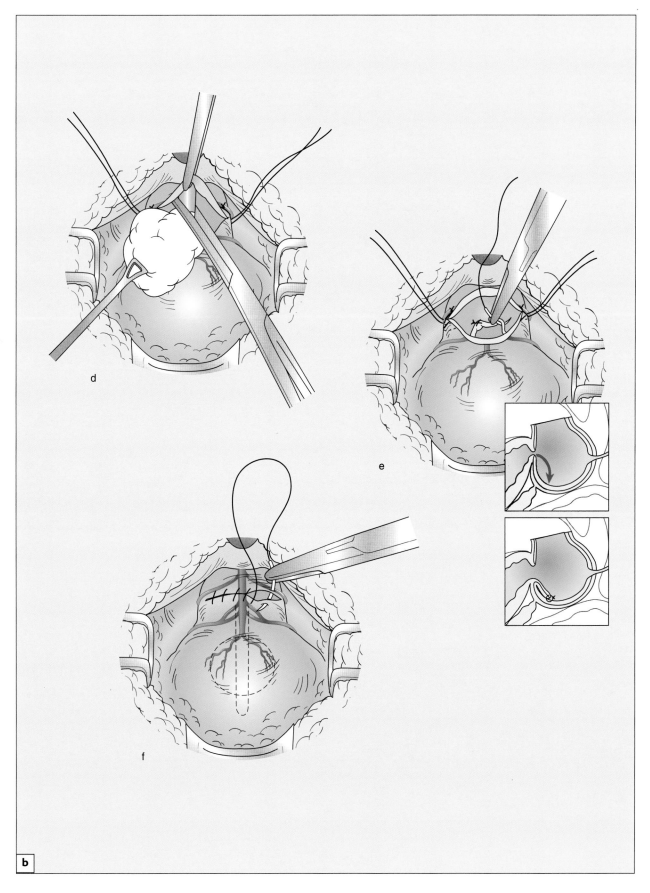

d

e

f

Figure 130   *Continued*

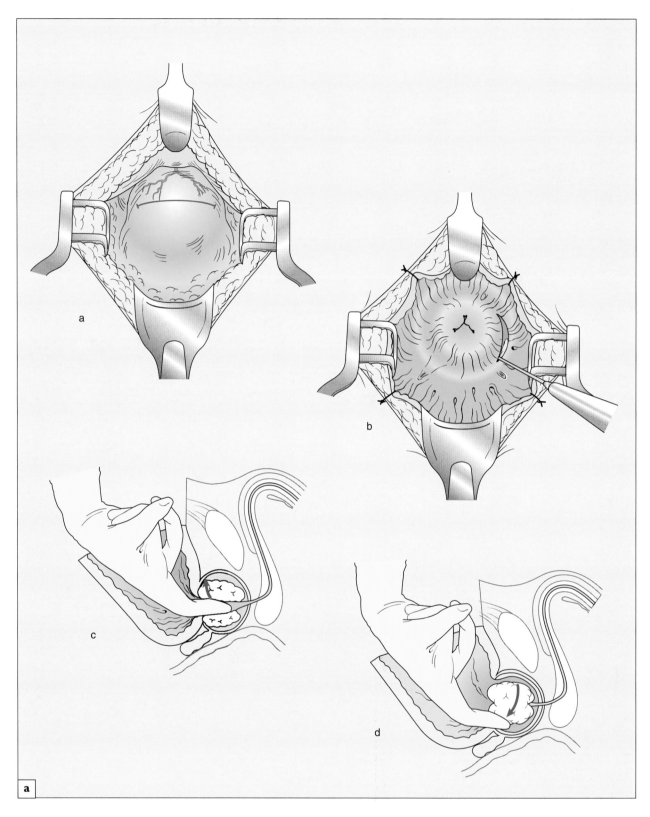

Figure 131   Transvesical prostatectomy: the bladder and anterior prostate are exposed through a transverse lower abdominal incision (a). The bladder is opened and the epithelium over the prostate incised (b). The adenoma involving the transitional zone is then enucleated ((c) and (d)). The attachment to the distal sphincter is divided with scissors (e). The bladder neck is advanced into the prostate cavity (f) and sutured posteriorly (g). A catheter is placed and the bladder neck reconstructed with interrupted sutures. Finally, the bladder is closed in two layers (h) (*continued*)

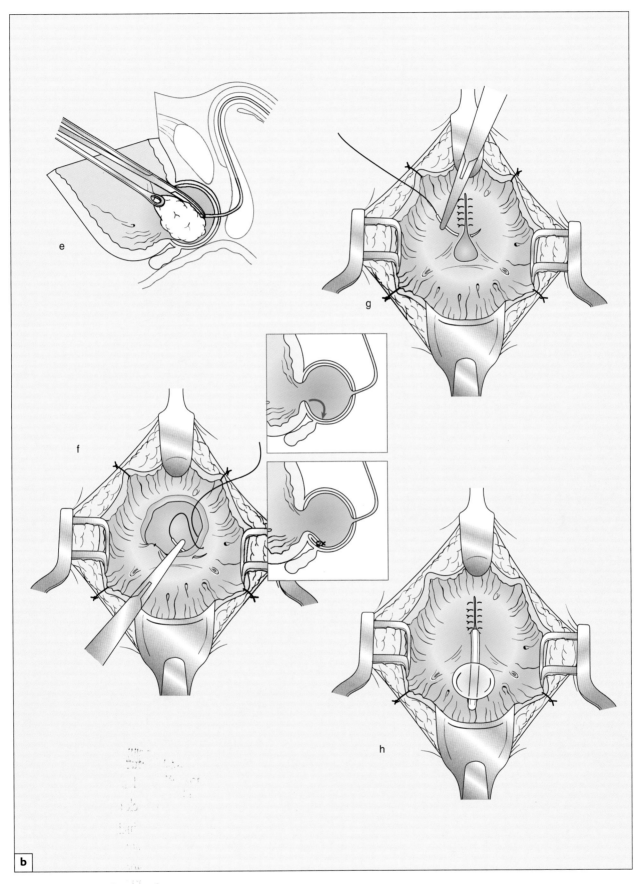

Figure 131 *Continued*

PROSTATE CANCER

Chemoprevention

The prospects for chemoprevention of prostate cancer currently look promising[73]. A large trial is underway examining the role of vitamin E and selenium. The new dual 5α-reductase inhibitor dutasteride may also have a role in this respect on the basis of early placebo-controlled data (Figure 134).

Early disease

The management of early prostate cancer is one of the most controversial areas of prostate disease, and is likely to remain so until the results of several randomized controlled trials currently underway become available[74]. A Scandinavian trial comparing radical prostatectomy with external beam radiotherapy with watchful waiting has recently been reported[75]. This study has confirmed that radical prostatectomy can reduce prostate cancer-specific mortality, but, perhaps because of the relatively high mean age (64.2 years) and consequent co-morbidity rate of subjects included in this study, as well as the relatively short follow-up, there is not as yet a reduction in overall mortality, although this is likely to become evident during further follow-up. The US-based PIVOT trial comparing radical prostatectomy with watchful waiting is now fully recruited with younger, fitter and lower-stage patients, but the results will not be available for some years.

Patients with clinically localized prostate cancer (i.e. biopsy-proven disease with no evidence of extra-prostatic extension) should be informed about the advantages and disadvantages of the following treatment options:

(1) *Watchful waiting*: The option of active surveillance is most applicable in men with low-volume, less aggressive disease and in those with a life expectancy of less than 10 years. Regular PSA determinations are recommended and active treatment instituted if disease progression occurs.

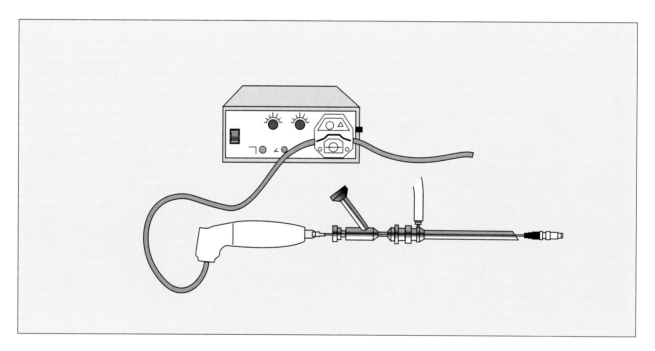

Figure 132   The Holmium laser (above) can be used for resection of the prostate with tissue morcellation. (a) An incision is made in the bladder neck at the 5 o'clock position. The incision is lengthened to the level of the verumontanum; (b) further incisions will be made at 7 o'clock, 1 o'clock and 11 o'clock positions; (c) the second incision is made at the 7 o'clock position; (d) the first two incisions are joined just proximal to the verumontanum; (e) if necessary, the median lobe can be divided into one or more pieces; (f) the lateral lobes are undermined; (g) the bladder neck incisions are then made at the 1 o'clock and 11 o'clock positions; (h) a combination of resection and/or vaporization can be used to eliminate any residual tissue (*continued*)

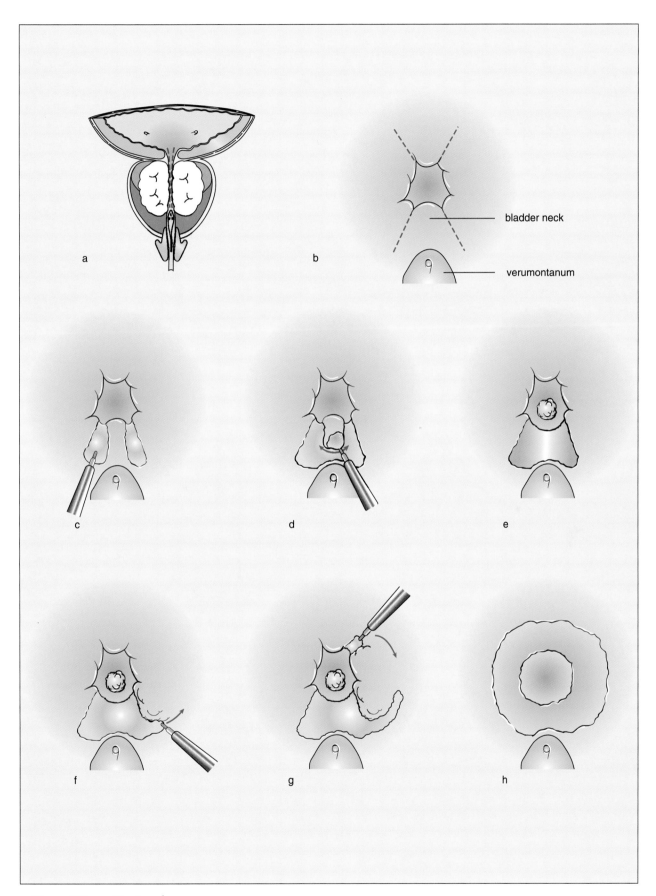

Figure 132 *Continued*

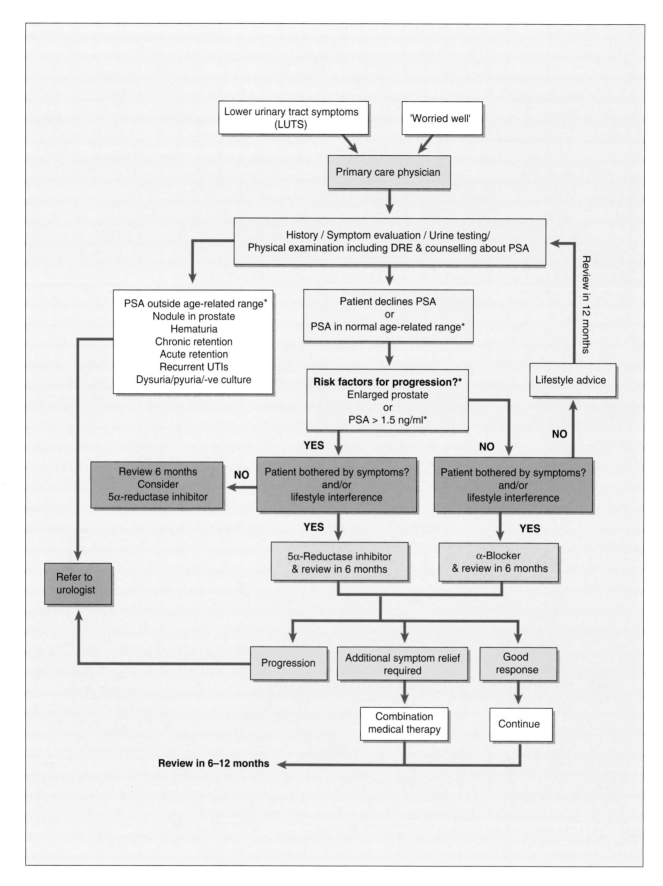

Figure 133   A proposed decision diagram for the management of benign prostatic hyperplasia-related lower urinary tract symptoms (LUTS) in primary care

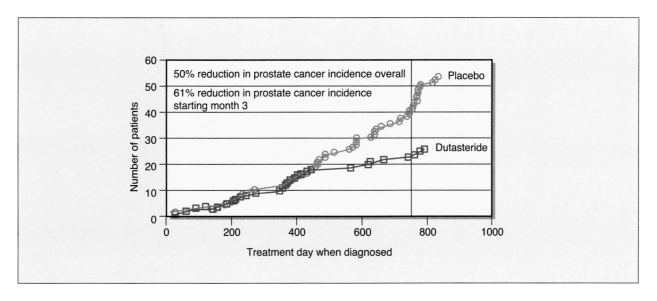

Figure 134   Possible chemopreventative action against prostate cancer by the dual 5α-reductase inhibitor dutasteride

(2) *Radical prostatectomy:* Considered by many to constitute the gold standard treatment, radical prostatectomy involves the removal of the entire prostate, either retropubically, perineally or laparoscopically (Figure 135). Provided that all cancer tissue is excised (i.e. all surgical margins, seminal vesicles and lymph nodes are clear), then life expectancy is equivalent to that of an age-matched individual who has never suffered cancer. Side-effects include a low risk (< 2–3%) of stress incontinence but a higher (> 50%) risk of erectile dysfunction, even when nerve-sparing techniques are employed. However, both these problems improve with time and can now be treated reasonably effectively. Provided that the entire prostate, including all cancer, has been excised, the serum PSA will fall to < 0.1 ng/ml postoperatively. This facilitates follow-up and permits early identification of tumor recurrence. Recently, laparoscopic radical prostatectomy has been developed (Figure 136) with reduced bleeding and shorter hospital stay. Robotic assistance is claimed to enhance potency and continence results[76] (Figure 137).

(3) *External beam radiotherapy:* External beam radiotherapy (EBRT) can provide an effective form of therapy for early prostate cancer. Results have been enhanced by the use of neoadjuvant androgen ablation, usually with a LHRH analog [77]. Side-effects include proctitis and rectal bleeding due to inclusion of the anterior rectal wall in the treatment field. These can be reduced by the use of conformal technology, which focuses treatment more accurately on the prostate.

(4) *Brachytherapy:* Brachytherapy involves the transperineal implantation of radioactive seeds into the prostate under light anesthesia (Figure 138). Swelling of the gland in response may cause a worsening of lower urinary tract symptoms for some time. Thus, this form of treatment should be used with caution in patients with pre-existing severe bladder outflow obstruction. In patients who are considered at higher risk of recurrence, brachytherapy may be used in combination with EBRT, although caution must be exercised with regards to the overall radiation dosage. Brachytherapy cannot be used in men who have previously undergone transurethral resection of the prostate because the seeds are not retained satisfactorily[78].

(5) *Cryotherapy:* So-called third-generation cryotherapy involves insertion of between ten and 20 needles into the prostate and the creation of an ice ball within the gland. The method is currently growing in popularity and allows for retreatment, but for now should still be regarded as experimental (Figure 139)[79].

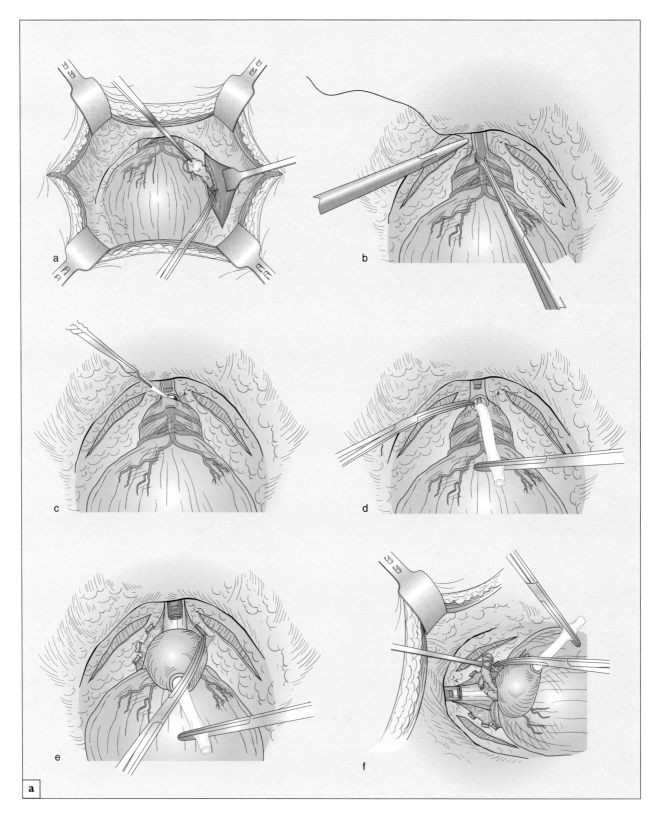

Figure 135   Open retropubic radical prostatectomy: (a) the obturator lymph nodes are dissected; (b) the dorsal vein complex is 'bunched' and sutured; (c) the dorsal vein and anterior urethra are divided; (d) the catheter is divided and the posterior wall of the urethra incised; (e) the lateral pedicles are secured; (f) the vasa are divided and the seminal vesicles dissected free; (g) the posterior dissection frees the prostate from the trigone; (h) the bladder neck is dissected away from the prostate; (i) an anastomosis is created over an 18F catheter (*continued*)

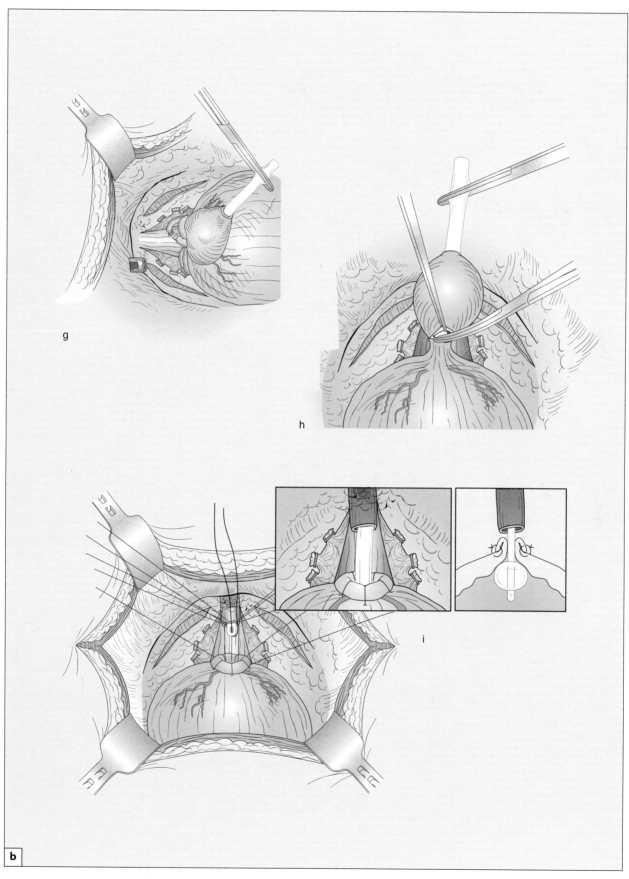

g

h

i

b

Figure 135 *Continued*

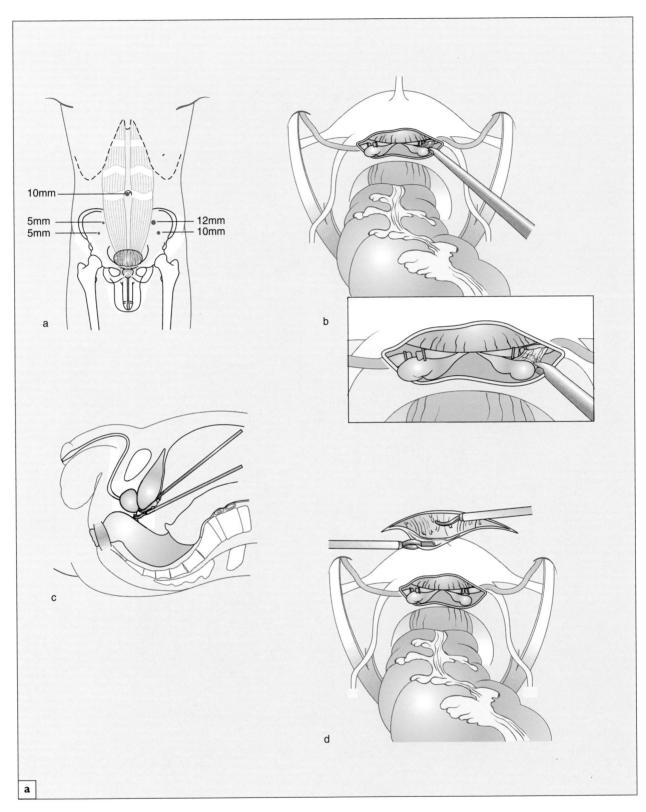

Figure 136   Laparoscopic radical prostatectomy: (a) five ports are inserted in fan array; (b) a transverse peritoneotomy in the retrovesical cul-de-sac exposes the vas deferens and seminal vesicles; (c) Denonvilliers'
fascia is incised horizontally; (d) the bladder is distended with saline and a peritoneotomy is made to
develop the space of Retzius; (e) the endopelvic fascia is incised bilaterally and the dorsal venous
complex secured; (f) the lateral pedicles are secured with staples; (g) an anastomosis is created over an
18F catheter (*continued*)

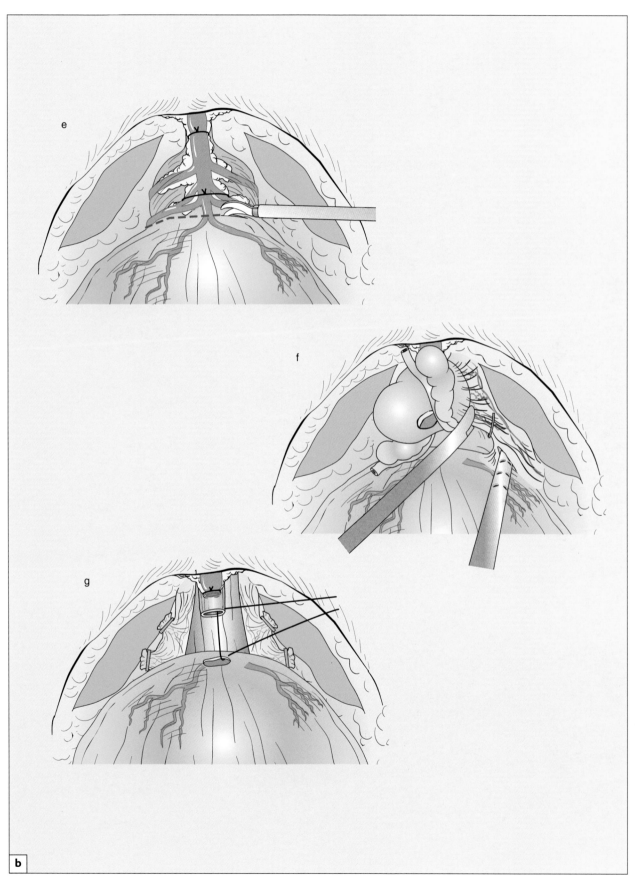

Figure 136   *Continued*

Antiandrogen monotherapy for those considered at high risk of recurrence

A group of patients who are treated with curative intent with either surgery or radiotherapy are considered as being at high risk of disease recurrence. These men present with higher PSA values, less well-differentiated cancers, and scans suggestive of extra-prostatic extension. Those undergoing surgery are often found to have positive surgical margins or involved seminal vesicles. Recent data[80] from a randomized study involving 8113 patients suggest that treatment with the antiandrogen bicalutamide at a dose of 150 mg/day can reduce the risk of objective disease progression by 42%. The main reported side-effects in the bicalutamide-treated patients were breast pain and gynecomastia.

Management of local recurrence

Unfortunately, a proportion of men treated by any of the above methods of curative intent eventually

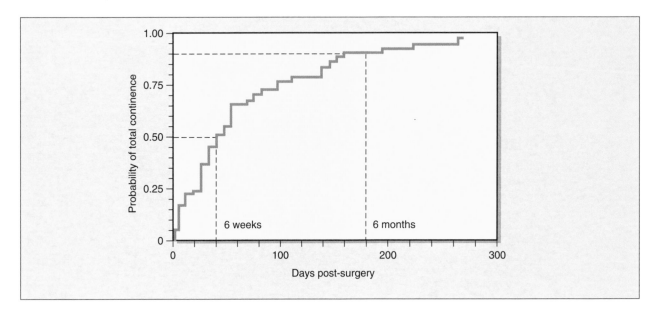

Figure 137   Continence after robotically assisted laparoscopic radical prostatectomy. Eventually, almost every patient regains continence, although this can take some time to occur[76]

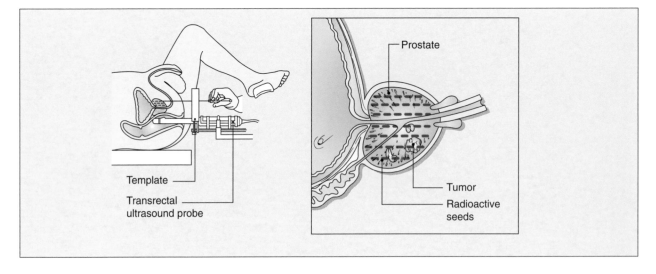

Figure 138   Brachytherapy: under ultrasound-guided control, radioactive seeds are placed within the prostate using a specially designed applicator grid

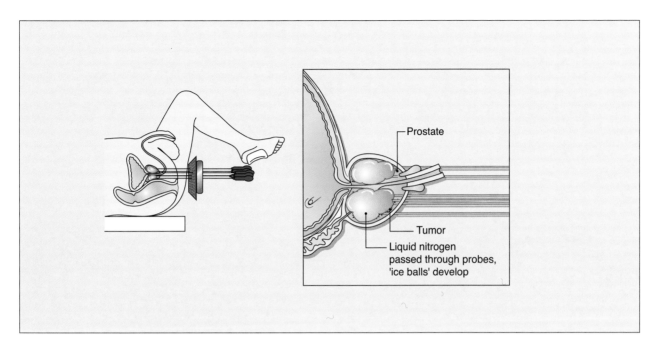

Figure 139   Cryotherapy: under ultrasound guidance, cooling needles are placed into the prostate and an ice ball created that destroys the tumor. Urethral sparing is achieved by a warming catheter

develop biochemical evidence of a progressive PSA rise. This is almost always an indicator of disease recurrence, but the exact localization of the residual or recurrent disease can be difficult. The longer the interval between initial treatment and subsequent PSA elevation, the more likely it is that the disease is local, rather than metastatic. TRUS-guided prostate biopsy, MRI scanning and bone scans are often negative. Immunoscintography using the prostate membrane specific antigen (PSMA)-based 'Prostascint' scan has low sensitivity and specificity. Histopathological interpretation of prostate biopsies after radiation therapy can be misleading, due to difficulties of interpretation (Figure 140).

Treatment will depend on the primary therapeutic modality employed. Radiation to the prostate bed can be used after radical prostatectomy with little additional morbidity. Salvage radical prostatectomy after either EBRT or brachytherapy carries a significant risk of incontinence, rectal injury and other morbidity. In these circumstances, androgen ablation is often the safer option, either with an antiandrogen or an LHRH analog. Cryotherapy (Figure 139) may be applicable in some cases but, at present, should be regarded as investigational. High-intensity focused ultrasound can also be employed in this context but there is limited experience (Figure 141).

Advanced disease and the role of LHRH analogs

Patients with prostate cancer involving lymph nodes, other soft tissues or the bony skeleton are described as suffering from advanced disease. In either circumstance, cure is not possible; however, androgen withdrawal with, for example, LHRH analogs will, in most cases, result in a remission that is maintained for, on average, 24–36 months, depending on the extent of the metastatic burden at presentation. Androgen ablation can be achieved either by bilateral orchidectomy or the use of depot LHRH analogs. Anti-androgens, such as bicalutamide, preserve some aspects of sexual function, but are not as effective in maintaining remission as the previously mentioned forms of androgen withdrawal when either bone or soft tissue metastases are present[80].

Hormone-independent prostate cancer

Eventually, as a result of the selection of androgen-independent clones of cancer cells, prostate cancer sufferers treated by androgen ablation suffer disease relapse. In this situation, the first step is to withdraw any anti-androgen, as this may result in a clinical remission and a transient improvement of PSA

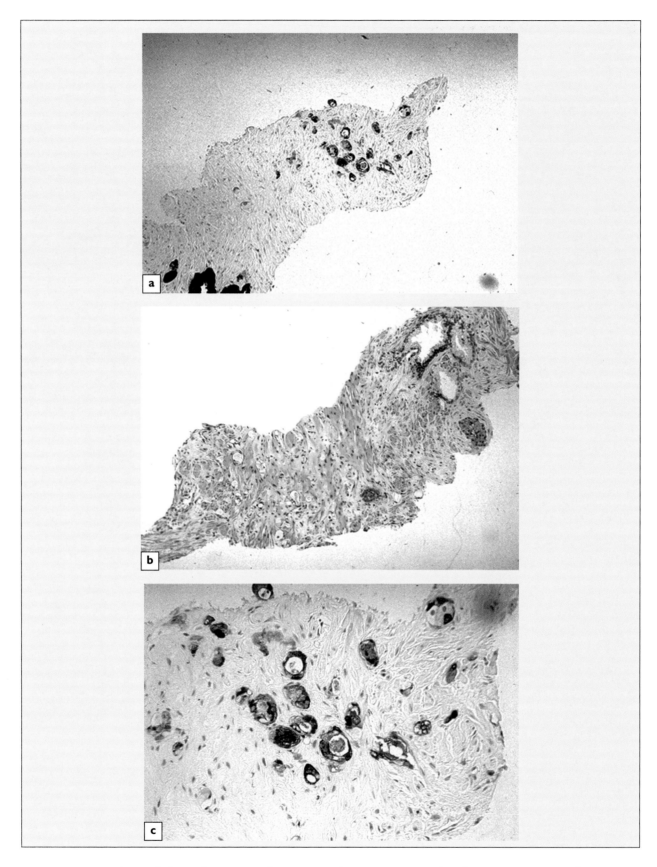

Figure 140   Histopathology of patients with recurrent adenocarcinomas within the prostate in spite of previous radiation therapy. The artefacts caused by irradiation changes can make histopathological interpretation difficult

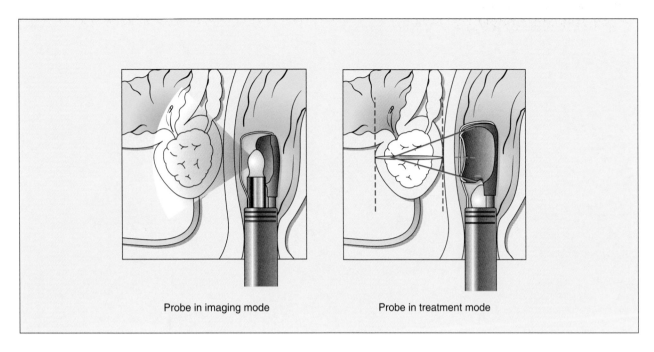

Probe in imaging mode   Probe in treatment mode

Figure 141   High-intensity focused ultrasound allows preliminary three-dimensional imaging of the prostate and subsequent targeted treatment by local heat generated by the precise focusing of high-intensity ultrasound waves under real-time monitoring

values. Second-line treatments include the use of oral estrogens in combination with either aspirin or intravenous chemotherapy. Recent data suggest that docetaxel (Taxotere), a microtubule inhibitor, may have a role in this respect, either as monotherapy or in combination, although phase III data are awaited to confirm this[81]. Other effective chemotherapy regimens include mitozantrone and estracyt, but only the latter currently has a license for use in this situation. Remissions are unfortunately relatively short-lived, but several newer approaches, including the use of tyrosine kinase inhibitors, and angiogenesis inhibitors are currently under investigation. Another new approach is the use of ET-1 antagonists.

The endothelin family of peptides has recently been identified as contributing significantly to the pathophysiology of prostate cancer[82]. In the normal prostate, ET-1 is produced by epithelial cells and appears in high concentrations in seminal fluid[83]. In prostate cancer, key components of the ET-1 clearance pathway, the endothelin-B (ET_B) receptors, and the degradative enzyme neutral endopeptidase are diminished, resulting in an increase in local ET-1 concentrations. Expression of the endothelin-A (ET_A) receptor also increases with tumor grade and stage.

There are multiple pathways by which the ET-1/ET_A axis may promote prostate cancer progression (*see* Figure 25). ET-1 is a mitogen for prostate cancer cell lines, and also for osteoblasts, the cell type which is pivotal in the hallmark osteoblastic response of bone to metastatic prostate cancer.

In a recent placebo-controlled study of the endothelin-A receptor antagonist atrasentan[84] (Figure 142) in 288 patients with hormone-refractory prostate cancer, the median time to progression was significantly prolonged (Figure 143) and time to PSA progression doubled (Figure 144). Side-effects included headache, peripheral edema and rhinitis, typically of mild to moderate severity.

Bisphosphonates have proven to be effective inhibitors of bone resorption, particularly when given intravenously. These compounds accumulate in the mineralized bone matrix, making it more resistant to dissolution by osteoclasts. Bisphosphonates are released during the process of bone resorption and are internalized by osteoclasts, reducing their activity and survival. This effect of osteoclast apoptosis is a result of the ability of nitrogen-containing bisphosphonates to inhibit the prenylation of GTPases (primarily farnesylation of Ras)[85] (Figures 145–147). A recent study of the bisphosphonate zoledronic acid[86] at a dose of 4 mg reported a

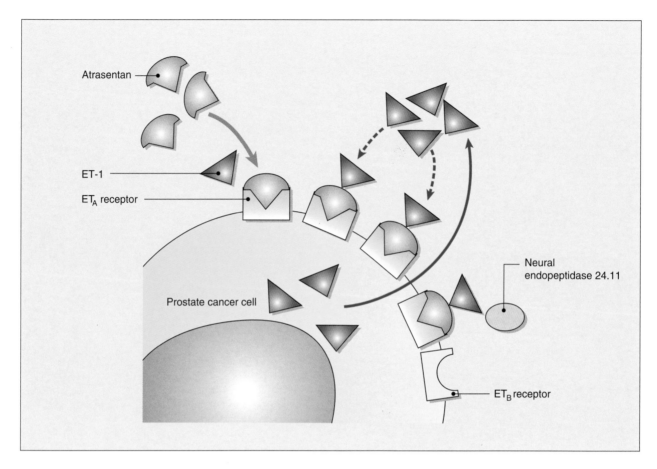

Figure 142   Prostate cancer is characterized by over-expression of both ET-1 and of the ET_A receptor. In contrast, the ET_B receptor, which predominates in normal cells, is present in low levels. Atrasentan is an orally available, specific and potent ET_A receptor antagonist

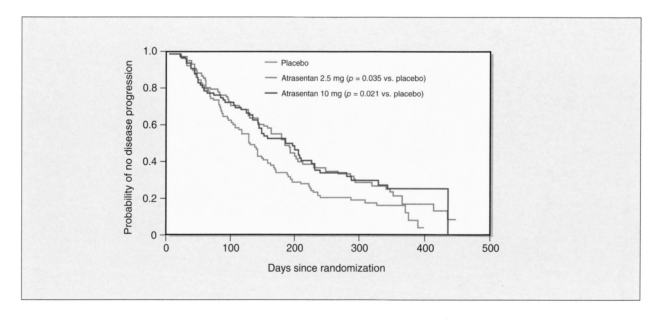

Figure 143   In the evaluable subset of patients with hormone-refractory prostate cancer, time to disease progression was significantly prolonged in the atrasentan 10 mg group compared with placebo (196 days vs. 129 days, respectively) ($p = 0.021$)

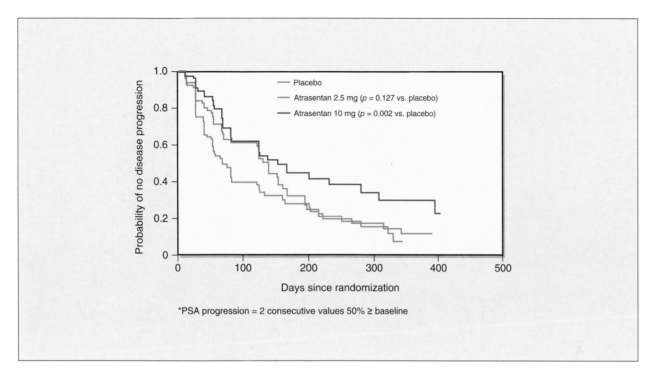

Figure 144   Atrasentan has also been shown to delay time to PSA progression in patients with metastatic hormone-resistant prostate cancer. In the evaluable subset of patients in the phase II study, median time to PSA progression was significantly greater in the group receiving atrasentan 10 mg compared with those receiving placebo (155 days vs. 71 days, respectively, $p = 0.002$)

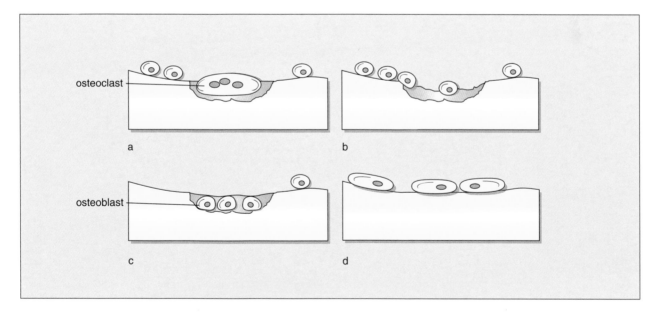

Figure 145   Normal bone remodelling. (a) Resorption: stimulated bone-lining cells (osteoblast precursors) release factors that bind to osteoclast receptors, leading to osteoclast differentiation and activity. Osteoclasts remove bone mineral and matrix, creating an erosion cavity. (b) Reversal: mononuclear cells prepare the bone surface for new osteoblasts to begin building bone. (c) Formation: successive waves of osteoblasts synthesize an organic matrix to replace resorbed bone and fill the cavity. (d) Resting: the bone surface is covered with flattened lining cells

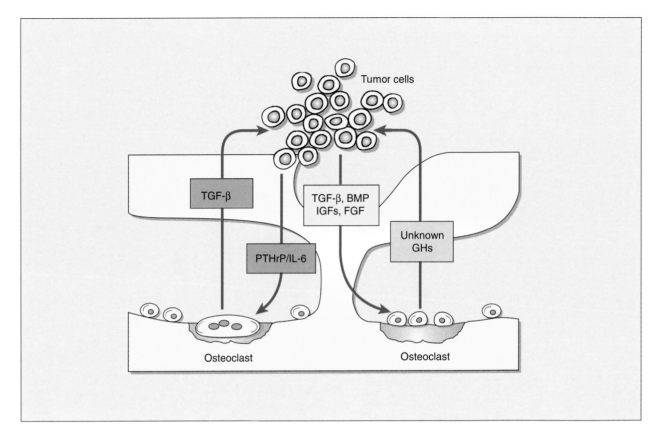

Figure 146   Imbalance of bone remodelling by prostate cancer cells and stimulation of metastases by locally released growth factors

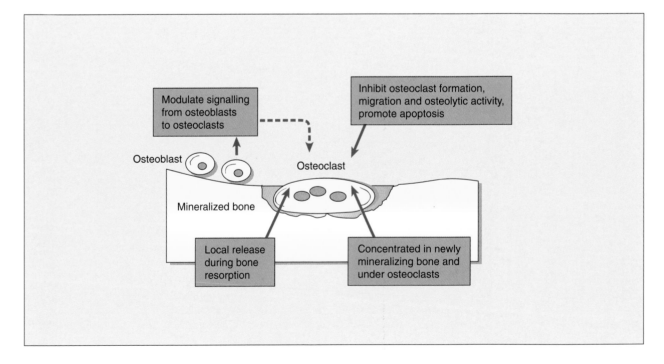

Figure 147   Bisphosphonates inhibit osteoclast formation and activity and promote apoptosis

significant (22%) reduction in the number of patients with a skeletal event compared with placebo (Figure 148) and a delay in the development of the first skeletal event (Figure 149). Zoledronic acid given as a 15-min infusion was well tolerated (Figure 150). Bisphosphonates work by inhibiting the osteoclasts associated with metastatic deposits. Local irradiation may produce useful palliation, as may the use of corticosteroids. When local complications, such as spinal cord compression, occur, surgical

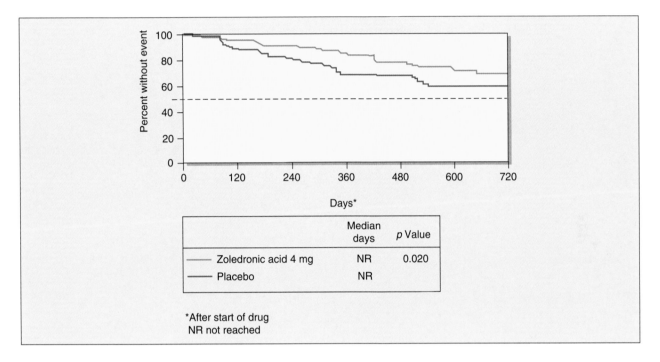

Figure 148   The bisphosphonate zoledronic acid significantly reduces the incidence of skeletal events in patients with metastatic prostate cancer

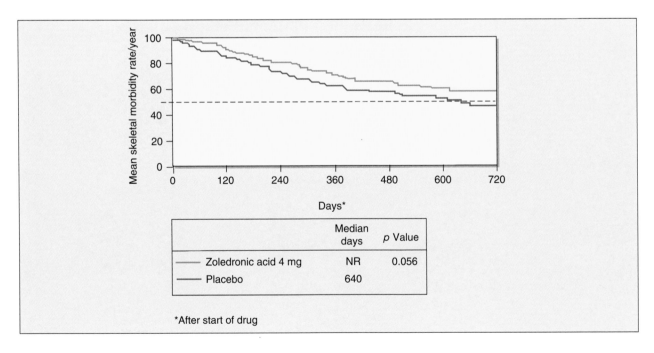

Figure 149   The bisphosphonate zoledronic acid significantly increases the time to first radiation for skeletal pain in men with metastatic prostate cancer

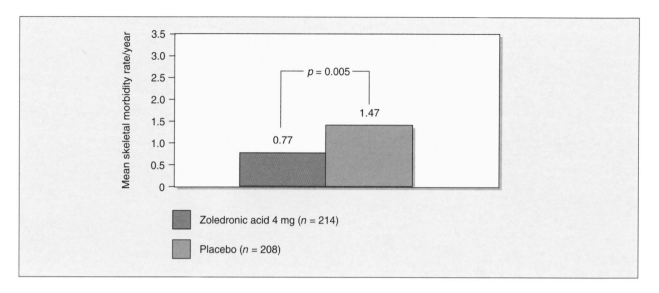

Figure 150   The bisphosphonate zoledronic acid significantly increases the time to first pathological fracture in men with metastatic prostate cancer

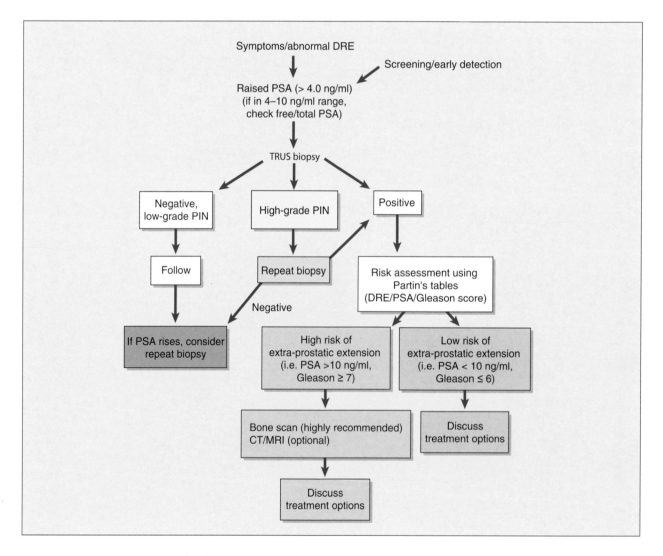

Figure 151   Decision tree for the management of early prostate cancer

decompression may be urgently required. The advise of the palliative care team should be sought in the management of cases of advanced hormone-refractory prostate cancer.

Decision diagrams for the management of localized, locally advanced and hormone-independent prostate cancer are shown in Figures 151–153.

PROSTATITIS

Unfortunately for the sufferers, the treatment of prostatitis remains somewhat unsatisfactory. In the presence of documented prostatic infection, treatment with antibiotics is logical, and these may need to be continued for 6 weeks or longer. Even if expressed prostatic secretions are negative, a response to antibiotics may be seen, especially if these are used in combination with anti-inflammatory agents. When an acute prostatic abscess is present, this may need to be drained transurethrally, and the pus cultured to determine appropriate antibiotic sensitivities. Chronic prostatitis has a very marked tendency to relapse, and patients should be

informed of this and counselled that further courses of treatment may become necessary. Currently, there is no convincing evidence that any invasive procedure, such as transurethral resection of the prostate or thermotherapy, is effective in treating or preventing recurrence of chronic prostatitis. A decision diagram for the management of prostatitis is shown in Figure 154.

SEXUAL FUNCTION AND THE PROSTATE

As the prostate and seminal vesicles are intimately involved in semen production, storage and ejaculation, it is not surprising that prostatic diseases and their treatments not uncommonly have a negative impact on sexual function. As mentioned, medical treatments for benign prostatic hyperplasia, especially tamsulosin, may cause retrograde ejaculation, while 5α-reductase inhibitors may produce loss of libido and erectile dysfunction. These effects are reversible on cessation of therapy[87]. Transurethral resection of the prostate is associated with retrograde ejaculation in more than two-thirds of cases; recent

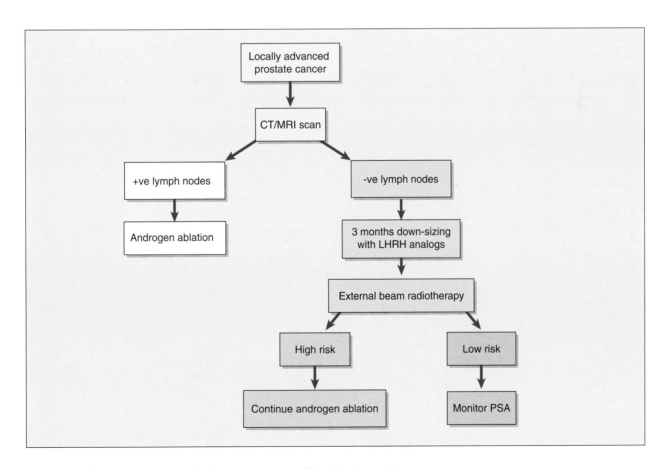

Figure 152   Decision tree for the management of locally advanced prostate cancer

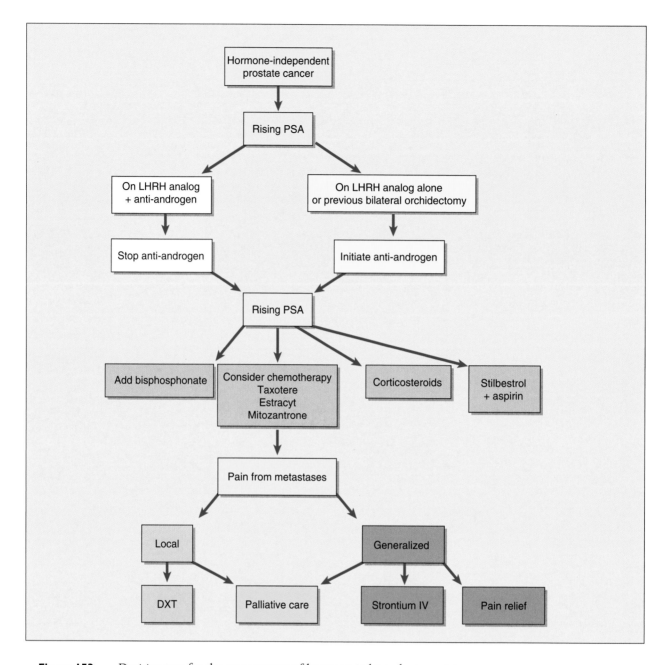

Figure 153 Decision tree for the management of hormone-independent prostate cancer

data, however, suggest that both α-blockers and transurethral resection of the prostate may improve overall sexual function, perhaps by virtue of their beneficial effect on other aspects of quality of life and other activities of daily living.

Treatments for localized prostate cancer are almost all associated with an incidence of erectile dysfunction. Androgen ablation, by whichever means, frequently causes loss of libido and erectile failure, but anti-androgens are less potent in this respect than the LHRH analogs[88].

Modern treatment for sexual dysfunction associated with prostatic disease includes the use of medical therapy with phosphodiesterase type 5 inhibitors such as sildenafil, vardenafil or tadalafil[89,90] (Figure 155). Apomorphine may also be effective[91]. Prostaglandin can be administered either transurethrally[92] or by intracavernosal injection (Figure 156). Vacuum devices can be useful in some patients; in others, the implantation of semirigid or inflatable penile prostheses offers the most cosmetic and effective solution (Figure 157).

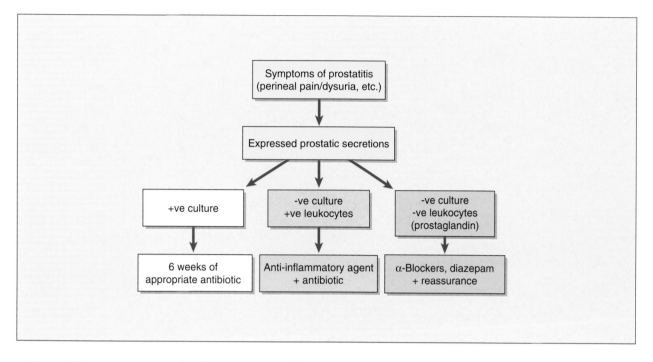

Figure 154   Decision tree for the management of prostatitis

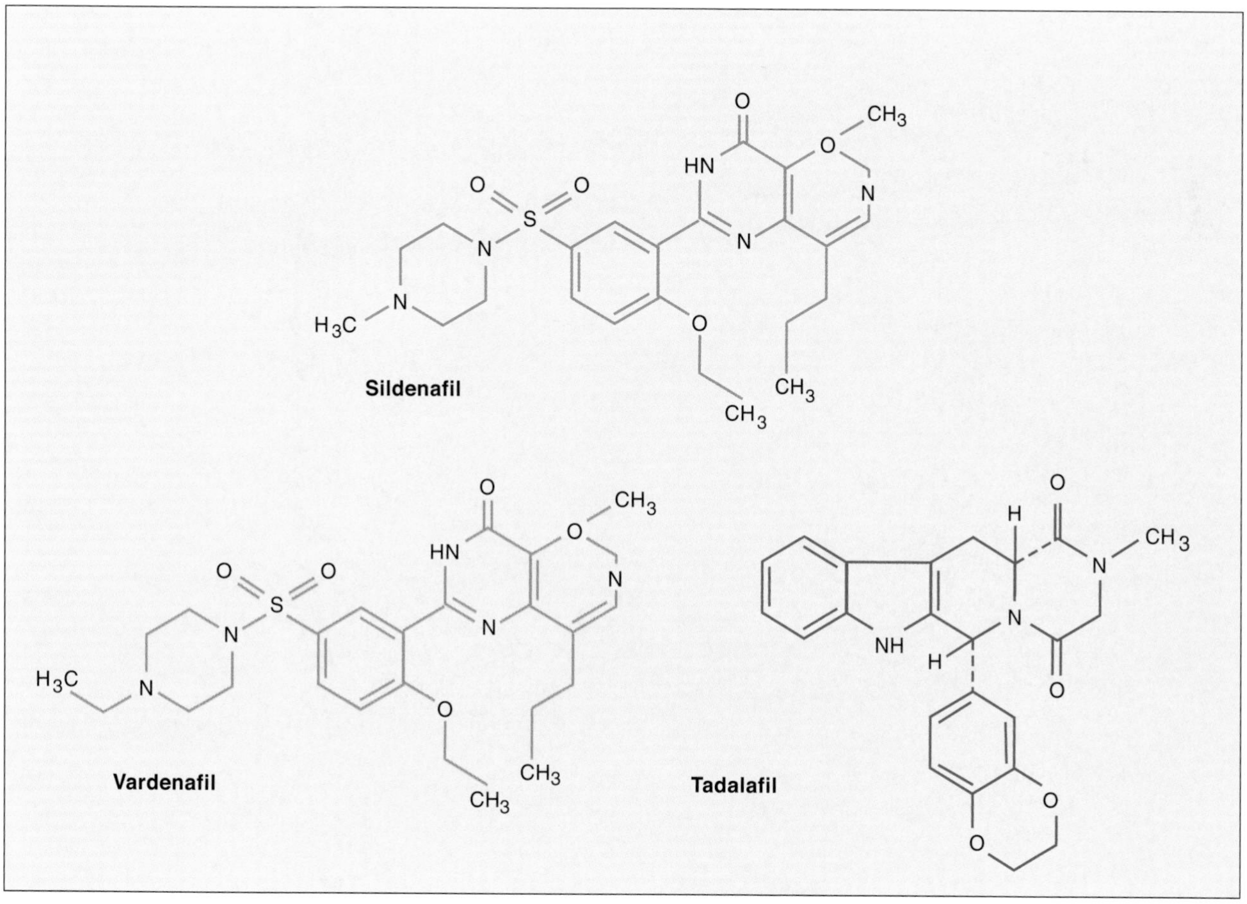

Figure 155   The chemical structures of sildenafil, vardenafil and tadalafil

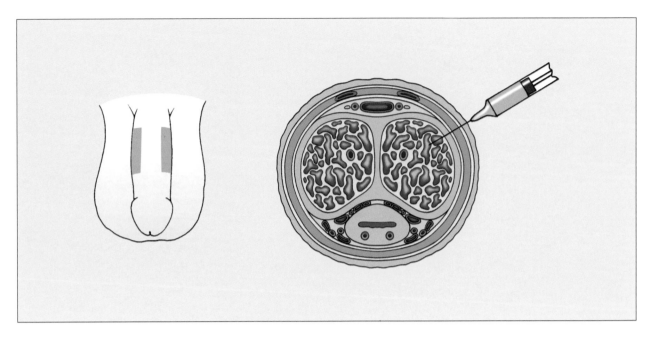

Figure 156   Intracavernous pharmacotherapy involves injection of vasoactive substances such as prostaglandin E_1, papaverine, phentolamine, or vasoactive intestinal polypeptide directly into the corpus cavernosum. An erection usually follows after 5–10 min and may last for up to 4 h

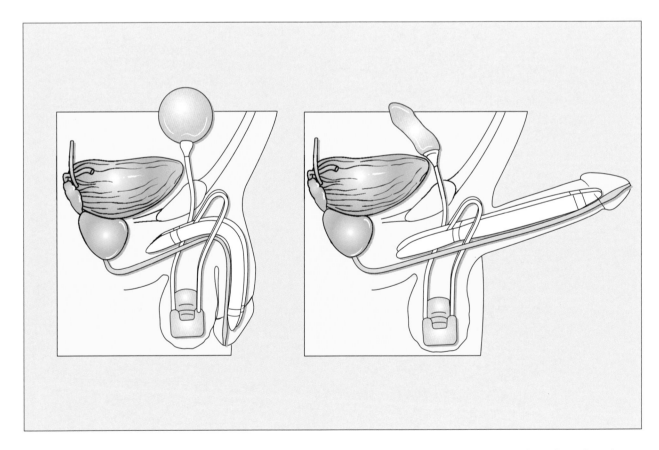

Figure 157   The three-component inflatable penile prosthesis produces a realistic erection and excellent flaccidity. Fluid is transferred from the reservoir to the cylinders to produce rigidity

19

Concluding perspectives

Recently, the prostate and the diseases to which it is so prone seem to have come to the forefront. The level of public interest has risen swiftly and with it the opportunities for research funding. This, in tandem with the recent explosive development of molecular biology, has produced new insights into the causes of benign prostatic hyperplasia, prostate cancer and prostatitis. For example, a hereditary factor in the pathogenesis of prostate cancer has been localized to a region of the long arm of chromosome 1[93]; this may account for the tendency for prostate cancer, like breast cancer, to run in certain families.

New consensus has now been reached concerning the diagnosis of prostatic diseases. PSA testing, although still controversial as a screening tool, is now established as a means of early detection, as well as staging. Ultrasound studies, guided biopsy and bone scans provide the cornerstone of the diagnosis of prostatic cancer. Biopsy confirmation is not usually required either for benign prostatic hyperplasia or prostatitis. Ultrasound studies and flow rate measurement usually suffice for the former, while culture of expressed prostatic secretions is indicated for prostatitis.

Benign prostatic hyperplasia therapy has seen a shift from surgery towards medical therapy. Both α-blockers[56] and 5α-reductase inhibitors appear safe and effective. The latter also have an important preventative effect[57]. A combination of α-blocker and 5α-reductase inhibitor has recently been demonstrated to be the most effective means of reducing the risk of benign prostatic hyperplasia progression[60].

While treatment of advanced prostate cancer is generally agreed upon, therapy for localized prostate malignancy is much more controversial[74]. In the absence of firm evidence from randomized controlled trials, the best we can do at present is explain to patients the advantages and disadvantages of radical retropubic prostatectomy, radical radiotherapy, brachytherapy, cryotherapy or watchful waiting.

Although significant progress has been made in these disease areas, much work remains to be done to improve the quality of life of those who suffer from benign prostatic hyperplasia and prostatitis, and to reduce significantly the death toll from prostate cancer. We also need to enhance the evidence base concerning the safety and effectiveness of the various competing treatment options. We can safely anticipate that the monumental effort currently being undertaken in many laboratories and clinics internationally will eventually translate into improvement of the outcomes for the many millions of prostate sufferers around the world.

References

1. Lowsley OS. The development of the human prostate gland with reference to the development of other structures of the neck of the urinary bladder. *Am J Anat* 1912;13:299

2. McNeal J. Regional morphology and pathology of the prostate. *Am J Clin Pathol* 1968;49:347–57

3. McNeal JE. The zonal anatomy of the prostate. *Prostate* 1891;2:35–49

4. Wang M, Valenzuela L, Murphy G, Chu T. Purification of human prostate specific antigen. *Invest Urol* 1979;17:159–63

5. Oesterling J. Prostate specific antigen: a critical assessment of the most useful tumor marker for adenocarcinoma of the prostate. *J Urol* 1991;145:907–23

6. Oesterling JE, Jacobsen SJ, Chute CG, *et al.* Serum prostate-specific antigen in a community-based population of healthy men. *J Am Med Assoc* 1993;270:860–4

7. Bartsch G, Muller H, Boerholzer M, Rohr H. Light microscopic stereological analysis of the normal human prostate and benign prostatic hyperplasia. *J Urol* 1979;122:487–91

8. Shapiro E, Hartanto V, Lepor H. Anti-desmin vs. anti-actin for quantifying the area density of prostatic smooth muscle. *Prostate* 1992;20:259–63

9. Lepor H, Gregerman M, Crosby M, Mostofi FK, Walsh PC. Precise localization of the autonomic nerves from the pelvic plexus to the corpora cavernosa: a detailed anatomical study of the adult male pelvis. *J Urol* 1985;133:207–12

10. Anderson KM, Liao S. Selective retention of dihydrotestosterone by prostatic nuclei. *Nature* 1968;219:277–9

11. Siiteri PK, Wilson JD. Dihydrotestosterone metabolism in prostate hypertrophy. 1. The formation of content of dihydrotestosterone in the hypertrophic prostate of man. *J Clin Invest* 1970;49:1737–45

12. Coffey DS. The endocrine control of normal and abnormal growth of the prostate. In *Urologic Endocrinology*. Philadelphia: WB Saunders, 1986:170–93

13. Ruffolo R, Nichols A, Stadel J, Hieble J. Structure and function of alpha adrenoceptors. *Pharm Rev* 1991;43:475–505

14. Schwinn DA, Lomasney JW, Lorenz WE. Molecular cloning and expression of the cDNA for a novel alpha-1 adrenergic receptor subtype. *J Biol Chem* 1990;265:8183–9

15. Zhau HE, Wan DS, Zhou J, Miller GJ, von Eschenbach AC. Expression of c-erb B-2/neu proto-oncogene in human prostatic cancer tissues and cell lines. *Mol Carc* 1992;5:320–7

16. Linehan WM. Molecular genetics of tumor suppressor genes in prostate carcinoma: the challenge and the promise ahead [Editorial]. *J Urol* 1992;147:808–9

17. Effert PJ, Neubauer A, Walther PJ, Liu ET. Alterations of the p53 gene are associated with the progression of a human prostate carcinoma. *J Urol* 1992;147:789–93

18. Bookstein R, Rio P, Madreperla SA, Hong FE. Promoter deletion and loss of retinoblastoma gene expression in human prostate carcinoma. *Proc Natl Acad Sci* 1990;87:7762–6

19. Hollstein M, Sidransky D, Vogelstein B, Harris B. p53 mutations in human cancers. *Science* 1991;253:49–53

20. Sarkar F, Sakr W, Li Y, Maloska JE. Analysis of retinoblastoma (RB) gene deletion in human prostatic carcinoma. *Prostate* 1992;21:145–52

21. Wakui S, Furusato M, Itoh T, *et al*. Tumor angiogenesis in prostatic carcinoma with and without bone marrow metastasis: a morphometric study. *J Pathol* 1992;168:257–62

22. Weidner N, Carrol PR, Flax JE. Tumor angio-genesis correlates with metastasis in invasive prostate carcinoma. *Am J Pathol* 1993;143:401–9

23. Kirby R, Lowe D, Bultitude M, Shuttleworth K. Intraprostatic urinary reflux: an aetiological factor in abacterial prostatitis. *Br J Urol* 1982;54:729–31

24. Bostwick D, Pacelli A, Lopez-Beltran A. Molecular biology of prostatic intraepithelial neoplasia. *Prostate* 1996;29:117–34

25. Bostwick DG. Premalignant lesions of the prostate. *Semin Diag Pathol* 1988;5:240–53

26. Bostwick DG, Brawer MK. Prostatic intraepithelial neoplasia and early invasion in prostate cancer. *Cancer* 1987;59:778–94

27. Gleason DF. Histologic grading and clinical staging of prostatic carcinoma. In Tannenbaum M, ed. *Urologic Pathology: The Prostate*. Philadelphia: Lea & Febiger, 1977:171–98

28. Brawer MK, Deering RE, Brown M, Preston SD, Bigler SA. Predictors of pathologic stage in prostatic carcinoma. The role of neovascularity. *Cancer* 1994;73:678–87

29. Sinha AA, Quast BJ, Wilson ML, *et al*. Prediction of pelvic lymph node metastasis by the ratio of cathepsin B to stefin A in patients with prostate carcinoma. *Cancer* 2002;94:3141–9

30. Berry SJ, Coffey DS, Walsh PC, Ewing LL. The development of human benign prostatic hyperplasia with age. *J Urol* 1984;132:474–9

31. Arrighi H, Guess H, Metter E, Fozard J. Symptoms and signs of prostatism as risk factors for prostatectomy. *Prostate* 1990;16:253–61

32. Drach GW, Layton TN, Binard WJ. Male peak urinary flow rate: relationship of volume voided and age. *J Urol* 1979;122:210–14

33. Roerhborn CG, McConnell J, Bonilla J, *et al*. Serum prostate specific antigen is a strong predictor of prostate growth in men with benign prostatic hyperplasia. *J Urol* 2000;163:13–20

34. Jacobsen SJ, Jacobsen DJ, Girman CJ, *et al*. Natural history of prostatism: risk factors for acute urinary retention. *J Urol* 1997;158:481–7

35. Goltzman D. Mechanisms of the development of osteoblastic metastases. *Cancer* 1997;80:1581–7

36. Mundy GR. Mechanisms of bone metastases. *Cancer* 1997;80:1546–56

37. Barry M, Fowler F, O'Leary M, *et al*. The American Urological Association symptom index for benign prostatic hyperplasia. *J Urol* 1992;148:1549–57

38. Barry M, Fowler F, O'Leary M, *et al*. Correlation of the American Urological Association symptom index with self-administered versions of the Madsen-Iversen, Boyarsky, and Maine Medical Assessment Program symptom indexes. *J Urol* 1992;148:1558–63

39. Chodak GW, Keller P, Schoenberg HW. Assessment of screening for prostate cancer using the digital rectal examination. *J Urol* 1989;141:1136–8

40. Catalona W, Smith D, Ratliff T, *et al*. Measurement of prostate specific antigen in serum as a screening test for prostate cancer. *N Engl J Med* 1991;324:1156–61

41. Catalona W, Richie J, Ahmann F, *et al*. A multicenter examination of PSA and digital rectal exam-ination for early detection of prostate cancer in 6,374 volunteers. *J Urol* 1993;149:412A

42. Lilja H, Christensson A, Dahlen U, *et al*. Prostate specific antigen in serum occurs predominantly in complex with alpha1 antichemotrypsin. *Clin Chem* 1991;37:1618–25

43. Dunsmuir W, Feneley M, Corry D, Bryan J, Kirby R. The day-to-day variation (test–retest reliability) of residual urine measurement. *Br J Urol* 1996;77:192–3

44. Feneley M, Dunsmuir W, Pearce J, Kirby RS. Reproducibility of uroflow measurement: experience during a double-blind, placebo-controlled study of doxazosin in benign prostatic hyperplasia. *Urology* 1996;47:658–63

45. Rickards D. Transrectal ultrasound. *Br J Urol* 1992;69:449–55

46. Rifkin M, Choi H. Implications of small, peripheral hypoechoic lesions in endorectal US of the prostate. *Radiology* 1988;166:619–22

47. Ohori M, Egawa S, Shinohara K, Wheeler T, Scardino P. Detection of microscopic extracapsular extension prior to radical prostatectomy for clinically localised prostate cancer. *Br J Urol* 1994;74:72–9

48. Wu CL, Carter HB, Naqibuddin M, et al. Effect of local anaesthesia on patient recovery after transrectal biopsy. *Urology* 2001;57:935–9

49. Hodhe KK, McNeal JE, Stamey TA. Ultrasound-guided transrectal core biopsies of the palpably abnormal prostate. *J Urol* 1989;142:66–70

50. Epstein JL, Walsh PC, Carter HB. Importance of posterolateral needle biopsies in the diagnosis of prostate cancer. *Urology* 2001;57:1112–16

51. Hricak H, Dooms C, Jeffery R, *et al.* Prostatic carcinoma assessment by clinical assess-ment, CT and MRI imaging. *Radiology* 1987;162:331–6

52. Chelsky MJ, Schnall MD, Seidmon EJ, Pollack HM. Use of endorectal surface coil magnetic resonance imaging for local staging of prostate cancer. *J Urol* 1993;150:391–5

53. Jorgensen T, Muller C, Kaalhus O, Danielsen H, Tveter K. Extent of disease based on bone scan: Important prognostic indicator for patients with metastatic prostate cancer. *Eur Urol* 1995;28:40–6

54. Chybowski FM, Larson-Keller JJ, Bergstralh EJ, *et al.* Predicting radionuclide bone scan findings in patients with newly diagnosed, untreated prostate cancer. Prostate-specific antigen is superior to all other clinical parameters. *J Urol* 1991;145:313

55. Djavan B, Marberger M. A meta-analysis on the efficacy and tolerability of alpha-1 antagonists in patients with lower urinary tract symptoms suggestive of benign prostatic obstruction. *Eur Urol* 1999;36:1–13

56. Kirby RS. Doxazosin in benign prostatic hyperplasia: effects on blood pressure and urinary flow in normotensive and hypertensive men. *Urology* 1995;46:182–6

57. Kirby RS, Pool JL. Alpha adrenoceptor blockade in the treatment of benign prostatic hyperplasia: past, present and future. *Br J Urol* 1997;80:521–2

58. Ekman P. Maximum efficacy of finasteride is obtained within 6 months and maintained over 6 years. *Eur Urol* 1998;33:312–17

59. McConnell JD, Bruskewitz R, Walsh P, *et al.* The effect of finasteride on the risk of acute urinary retention and the need for surgical treatment among men with benign prostatic hyperplasia (PLESS). *N Engl J Med* 1998;338:557–63

60. McConnell JD. The long term effects of medical therapy in the progression of BPH: results from the MTOPS trial. *J Urol* 2002;167:1042

61. Roerhborn CG, Boyle P, Nickel JC, *et al.* Efficacy and safety of a dual inhibitor of 5alpha-reductase types 1 and 2 (dutasteride) in men with benign prostatic hyperplasia. *Urology* 2002;60:434–41

62. Roerhborn CG, Boyle P, Bergner D, *et al.* Serum prostate-specific antigen and prostate volume predict long-term changes in symptoms and flow rate: results of a four-year randomised trial comparing finasteride versus placebo. *Urology* 1999;54:662–9

63. Roerhborn CG, Malice M-P, Cook TJ, Girman CJ. Clinical predictors of spontaneous acute urinary retention in men with LUTS and clinical BPH: a comprehensive analysis of the placebo groups of several large clinical trials. *Urology* 2001;58:210–16

64. Boyle PA, Gould L, Roehrborn CG. Prostate volume predicts outcome of treatment of benign prostatic hyperplasia with finasteride: meta-analysis of randomised clinical trials. *Urology* 1996;48:398–405

65. Rosen R, O'Leary M, Altwein J, Kirby RS, *et al.* Lower urinary tract symptoms and male sexual dysfunction: the Multi-national Survey of the Aging Male (MSAM-7). *Lancet* 2003 (submitted)

66. Gormley GJ, Stoner E, Bruskewitz RC, *et al.* The effect of finasteride in men with benign prostatic hyperplasia. *N Engl J Med* 1992;327:1185–91

67. Hofner K, Jonas U. Alfuzosin: a clinically selective alpha blocker. *World J Urol* 2002;19:405–12

68. Lepor H. Long-term evaluation of tamsulosin in benign prostatic hyperplasia: placebo-controlled, double-blind extension of phase III trial. Tamsulosin Investigator Group. *Urology* 1998;51:901–6

69. Flannigan RC, Reda DJ, Wason, *et al.* Five year outcome of surgical resection and watchful waiting for men with moderately symptomatic benign prostatic hyperplasia: a Department of Veterans Affairs cooperative study. *J Urol* 1998;160:12–16

70. Gilling PJ, Mackey M, Cresswell M, *et al.* Holmium laser versus transurethral resection of the prostate: randomised prospective trial with at least 1 year follow-up. *J Urol* 1999;162:1640–4

71. Brookes ST, Donovan JL, Peters TJ, *et al.* Sexual dysfunction in men after treatment for lower urinary tract symptoms: evidence from randomised controlled trial. *BMJ* 2002;324:1059–61

72. Kashif KM, Foley SJ, Basketter V, Holmes SAV. Haematuria associated with BPH – natural history and a new treatment option. *Prostate Cancer and Prostatic Diseases* 1998;1:154–6

73. Fitzpatrick JM. Chemoprevention for prostate cancer – the way forward. *BJUI* 2003;91:589–94

74. Kirby RS. Treatment options for early prostate cancer. *Urology* 1998;52:948–62

75. Holmberg l, Bill-Axelson A, Helgesen F, *et al.* A randomised trial comparing radical prostatectomy with watchful waiting in early prostate cancer. *N Engl J Med* 2002;347:781–9

76. Tewari A, Peabody J, Sarle R, *et al.* Technique of Da Vinci robot-assisted anatomic radical prostatectomy. *Urology* 2002;60:569–72

77. Bolla M, Collette L, Blank L, *et al.* Long-term results with immediate androgen suppression and external irradiation in patients with locally advanced prostate cancer (an EORTC study): a phase III randomised trial. *Lancet* 2002;360:103–8

78. Ragde H, Elgamal A, Snow PB, *et al.* Ten year disease free survival after transperineal sonography-guided Iodine 125 brachytherapy with or without 45 Gray external beam irradiation in the treatment of patients with clinically localised, low to high Gleason grade prostate carcinoma. *Cancer* 1998;83:989–1001

79. Donnelly BJ, Saliken JC, Ernst DS, *et al.* Prospective trial of cryosurgical ablation of the prostate: 5 year results. *Urology* 2002;60:645–9

80. See WA, Wirth MP, McLeod DG, *et al.* Bicalutamide as immediate therapy either alone or as an adjuvant to standard care of patients with localised or locally advanced prostate cancer: first analysis of the early prostate cancer programme. *J Urol* 2002;168: 429–35

81. Beer TM, Eilers KM, Garzetto M, *et al.* Weekly high-dose calcitrol and docetaxel in metastatic androgen-independent prostate cancer. *J Clin Oncol* 2003;21: 123–8

82. Nelson JB, Halahi S, Conaway M, *et al.* Identification of endothelin-1 in the pathophysiology of metastatic adenocarcinoma of the prostate. *Nat Med* 1995;1: 944–9

83. Nelson JB, Carducci MA. The role of the endothelin axis in prostate cancer. *Prostate* 1999;1:495–9

84. Carducci MA, Padley RJ, Breul J, *et al.* Effect of endothelin-A receptor blockade with atrasentan on tumor progression in men with hormone-refractory prostate cancer: a randomised phase II placebo-controlled trial. *J Clin Oncol* 2003;21:679–89

85. Benford HL, Helfrich MH, Sehti S, *et al.* Inhibition of protein gerany/geranylation by bisphosphonates and CGT1298 causes activation of caspase 3-like proteases in osteoclasts. *Calcif Tissue Int* 1999;64 (Suppl):S45

86. Saad F, Gleason DM, Murray R, *et al.* A randomized, placebo-controlled trial of zoledronic acid in patients with hormone-refractory prostate carcinoma. *JNCI* 2002;94:1458–68

87. Kassabian VS. Sexual function in patients treated for benign prostatic hyperplasia. *Lancet* 2003;361:60–2

88. Fitzpatrick JM, Kirby RS, Krane RJ, *et al.* Sexual dysfunction associated with the management of prostate cancer. *Eur Urol* 1998;33:513–22

89. Carson CC, Burnett AL, Levine LA, *et al.* The efficacy of sildenafil citrate (Viagra) in clinical populations: an update. *Urology* 2002;60(Suppl 2):12–27

90. Padma-Nathan H, McMurray JG, Pullman WE, *et al.* On-demand IC351 (Cialis) enhances erectile function in patients with erectile dysfunction. *Int J Impot Res* 2001;13:2–9

91. Heaton JP. Characterising the benefit of apomorphine SL (Uprima) as an optimised treatment for representative populations with erectile dysfunction. *Int J Impot Res* 2001;(Suppl 13):S35–9

92. Padma-Nathan H, Hellstrom WJ, Kaiser FF, *et al.* Treatment of men with erectile dysfunction with transurethral alprostadil Medicated Urethral System for Erection (MUSE). *N Engl J Med* 1997;336:1–7

93. Smith JR, Freije D, Carpten JD, *et al.* Major susceptibility locus for prostate cancer on chromosome 1 suggested by genome-wide search. *Science* 1996;274:1371–5

Index